THE LE

Aubergine

KAREN PROTHEROE   **MOIRA VAN DER LINDE**

Contents

AUTHOR'S INTRODUCTION

Through my practice as a registered dietician, I have come to know many people like Sharon, whose story is outlined below. I realized that people needed not only *general guidelines* in terms of a healthy diet, but also *specific advice* on what exactly to eat to lose or maintain their weight. Most people know what they *should not* eat, but know very little about what they *should* eat. Eating involves much more than just consuming food.

SHARON'S STORY

At my wits' end after trying every conceivable diet, all of which cost me a fortune, I decided to see a dietician. I learnt a way of eating that was so normal, that I never really saw it as a 'diet', just as a new way of life for me and my family. I never made separate meals for my husband and four-year-old son – they ate the same healthy meals I ate. There was no weighing of food, no cutting out of certain food groups, no starving, no complicated charts to check the value of what we were eating, no headaches or lethargy – just staying away from FAT. I have learnt so much about FAT, and couldn't believe how much FAT I was 'innocently' consuming in so-called 'lite' meals and snacks. I now never buy a packet, box or tin of food without checking the FAT value. In six months I lost 17 kg, I have regained my self-confidence and I feel great about myself again. This is the only way to eat, and to stay healthy and trim.

A year later, Sharon is still maintaining her 17 kg weight loss, and finding it no trouble to do so. She has learnt what to buy, how to prepare food, how much to eat, and what to choose when faced with a choice of food outside the home. This book offers both general and specific advice for each of these areas: detailed low-fat shopping lists to guide you when you are shopping for food, general and specific tips for cooking and preparing food, tried and tested low-fat recipes, as well as a nationwide restaurant guide indicating low-fat menu options.

How to use the shopping lists:

- ❖ Check to see whether the food items you regularly buy appear in the shopping lists. If they are not listed, there is a good chance that they are not considered low-fat food items.
- ❖ If you are looking for a particular item, like a salad dressing, for example, use the Index to help you find the relevant listings. Then select a suitable salad dressing from the choices offered.
- ❖ Study the lists to see just how many food items are low in fat – this will help you choose a healthy, yet varied diet.

How to use the recipes:

- ❖ All the recipes are either straight from the kitchens of clients, friends, family or the authors themselves, and have all been successfully adapted to suit a low-fat lifestyle.
- ❖ By studying the recipes and seeing the principles applied, you will formulate ideas on how to adapt your own favourite recipes.

How to use the restaurant guide:

- ❖ Before going to a particular restaurant, look through the relevant chapter (pages 181–201) to find a discussion of a similar restaurant, and use this menu as a guideline. If you are going to a Thai restaurant, for example, use the guidelines set out for Wangthai.

AUTHOR'S ACKNOWLEDGEMENTS

I would like to thank the following people for either giving me their own tried and tested recipes, or for trying out my recipes and giving me valuable feedback: Colleen, Chanine, Tessa, Deidre, Barbara, June, Michelle v. G., Jean, Penny, Carol, Patsy, Marcia, Claudia, Liesl, Peta, Michelle Z., Colleen, Joan, Sharon, Janine, Pat, Cecily, Julia B., Andrée, Ingrid, Chris, Ananda, Robyn, Tanya, Peter and Debbie, Lorraine and Ferdi.

I would also like to say a big thank you to my contributing author, Moira, not just for all her hard work, but also for always being supportive. This book would not have happened without her expertise and enthusiasm. Moira has asked me to thank her parents, Ellen and Steve, and friends who have been a constant source of encouragement and support.

My thanks also go to the Health & Racquet Club for the opportunity to develop my practices in their clubs. A big thank you to Laura and Linda at Struik for their support and especially to Laura, for her expert and endless editing of the book. Julia Goedecke and Cecily Fuller were both kind enough to read through my work and give valid comments.

Last, but not least, I would like to thank my parents and Bron and Boris for always being there for me, to thank Mel for listening, and to thank Robert for inspiring me to write this book.

FOREWORD

It is seldom that a company has dominated an industry in the way in which the Health & Racquet Club has done in the field of health and fitness. As Scientific Advisor to the group, I feel privileged, therefore, to have been asked to write a foreword to a book that the Health & Racquet Club wishes to endorse.

Over the years I have worked professionally with Karen Protheroe within the health club environment. It is here that she operates her dietetic practices and she has, through ongoing interaction with her clients and club members, developed a unique understanding of their needs. And there is no doubt that this book was inspired by the many questions that her clients have asked her and the kind of help they have required. This book fulfils the needs of both the weight-conscious and the health-conscious.

To my knowledge *The Lean Aubergine* is the first book of its kind to offer an up-to-date listing of low-fat South African foods used for recipes, a low-fat shopping guide compiled with specific reference to products available in South African stores, and a low-fat menu guide referring to nationwide South African restaurants. This book is not about telling us that fats are bad, as most of us know this by now. Rather, it sets out to teach and guide us in making low-fat choices – whether we are buying or cooking food, or ordering dishes off a restaurant menu.

The Lean Aubergine is practical and simple to understand, yet original and inspiring. It takes the mystery out of following a balanced, sensible diet and deals effectively with the most contentious issues in dietetics today. In the broader context of health enhancement, it meets a vital need.

ROB COWLING
Scientific Advisor – Health & Racquet Club

CHAPTER ONE

Choosing a Low-Fat Lifestyle

INTRODUCTION

You may ask what exactly a low-fat lifestyle is, and why it is recommended. Surely we all know by now that to be healthy and to lose weight or to avoid gaining weight we need to cut down on the amount of fat we consume? Most of us know, for example, that we should, at the very least, be buying low-fat milk and avoiding fried foods. Through my practice as a Registered Dietician, however, I have come to realize that many people still have misconceptions about what constitutes healthy eating in terms of limiting their fat intake.

Many clients who come and see me tell me that they cannot understand why they are gaining weight, as they have cut all fats out of their diet. They tell me, for instance, that they have muesli instead of bacon and eggs for breakfast, eat rusks and digestive biscuits instead of normal biscuits, muffins instead of cake, use olive oil instead of sunflower oil, chicken instead of red meat, and so forth. Little do they realize, however, that many so-called 'health' foods contain hidden fats.

While we may easily be able to identify that butter, oil, cream and fried foods are high in fat, we may just as easily be misled by certain other foodstuffs. Did you know, for example, that a bowl of crunchy muesli or granola has almost the same fat content as bacon and eggs? Olive oil has the same fat content as any other oil, such as sunflower or canola oil. A rusk has the same fat content as two chocolate biscuits. Many health bars are higher in fat than a bar of chocolate – in fact, diabetic chocolate contains more fat than normal chocolate and a seed bar has double the fat of a small bag of potato crisps.

'Hidden' fats play a major role in weight gain and, in addition to this, these fats are often of a form that is unhealthy. This book aims to help you identify the hidden fats in food and, more importantly, shows you how to avoid unhealthy fats without resorting to extreme dietary measures.

AVERAGE DAY	FAT CONTENT (g)
Breakfast	
1 cup crunchy muesli	22.6
1 cup 2% milk	4.8
Mid-morning snack	
1 cup coffee with 2% milk and sweetener	1.4
1 muesli rusk	5
Lunch	
2 slices whole-wheat bread	1.5
cheese and margarine for sandwich	21.5
tomato for sandwich	0
1 small tub (175 ml) low-fat yoghurt	1.9
1 banana	0
Mid-afternoon snack	
2 cups home-made popcorn	7
2 cups coffee with 2% milk and sweetener	2.9
1 health bar e.g. yoghurt or seed bar	17.4
Supper	
90 g roast chicken	12.2
2 tbsp gravy	15.6
1 medium baked potato	0.1
butter on potato	8.2
cauliflower cheese	9.9
Greek salad with French dressing	19.3
¼ avocado	5.8
Evening snack	
3 bran biscuits	8.9
½ cup nuts	4.1
1 cup coffee with 2% milk and sweetener	1.4

TOTAL FAT CONTENT = 206.6 g (it should be approximately 40–70 g)

On the previous page I have analysed the average daily diet of someone who approached me for help, thinking that she was already following a low-fat diet. Note the hidden fats in muesli, a sandwich, popcorn, a health bar, gravy and dressed salads, and compare this to the very small amounts of fat in potatoes and bread, and nothing in bananas. The total fat content of this diet is approximately 200 g, whereas a healthy diet should contain only approximately 40–70 g of fat!

The above example illustrates how easily one can be misled, in terms of fat content, when trying to put together a successful eating plan – whether the aim is weight loss or merely a healthy diet. Many foodstuffs that seem to be 'slimming' or 'healthy' alternatives contain surprisingly large amounts of 'hidden' fat.

'FAT' TERMINOLOGY

It may be useful, at this point, to give brief explanations of some of the terms used when discussing fat.

BODY FAT

This is the amount of fat stored in the body; it can be represented as kilograms of fat or as a percentage of your total body weight. Body fat percentage is a useful tool when measuring weight loss, as it clearly distinguishes between the loss of fat and the loss of muscle weight. It may be noted here that muscle weighs more than fat. This explains why many people who embark on a balanced, low-fat diet in conjunction with an exercise program may initially gain weight. They may visibly be achieving a slimmer shape and losing fat weight, but they are building muscle weight.

BODY FAT DISTRIBUTION

Generally speaking, body fat distribution falls into one of two categories. Most women have a gynoid (pear-shaped) distribution of fat, which means that fat is stored mainly around the hips and thighs. Men are generally android (apple-shaped), and their fat is stored around the abdomen. An android fat distribution points to a risk for heart disease. Unfortunately, your body shape and pattern of fat distribution is often genetically determined and, although the size of the fat stores may change, the ultimate shape will remain the same.

CELLULITE

This term is used to refer to fat cells which are larger than normal, and found mainly on the buttocks and thighs. The cells are larger because they possess more storage potential than other fat cells. The presence of cellulite is, to a large extent, determined by gender and genetics.

DIETARY FATS

These can be broken up into several categories.

1. UNSATURATED FATS

Unsaturated fats may be either monounsaturated or polyunsaturated. Remember that excessive heating of unsaturated fats, which are normally considered beneficial to your health, can result in these fats becoming detrimental to your health.

Monounsaturated fats

The main sources of monounsaturated fats are olives and olive oil, canola oil, avocados, nuts and peanut oil. These fats have been found to contain properties which lower blood cholesterol.

Polyunsaturated fats

These fats are found in sunflower oil, soft margarines packaged in tubs, cod-liver oil, evening primrose oil, and oily fish such as mackerel, salmon and sardines. Polyunsaturated fats have more of a neutral effect on blood cholesterol levels and should be used in moderation.

2. SATURATED FATS

These fats are found in all animal products (e.g. meat, cheese, butter, cream, etc.) as well as in coconut and palm kernel oil. Saturated fats increase blood cholesterol levels and should therefore be avoided when-ever possible.

3. CHOLESTEROL

This wax-like substance, which is present in body tissues, is essential for normal functioning. The body makes all the cholesterol that it needs and, because cholesterol is also found in excess in our Western diet, the body can become oversupplied with cholesterol. This may result in an increase in cholesterol in the blood and arteries may even begin to become clogged up, which could result in a stroke or heart attack.

There are two main types of blood cholesterol, called LDL-cholesterol and HDL-cholesterol (LDL = low-density lipoprotein; and HDL = high-density lipoprotein). LDL-cholesterol is regarded as the 'bad cholesterol' that clogs up arteries, while HDL-cholesterol is the 'good cholesterol' that carries the cholesterol away from the arteries back to the liver, where it is broken down to be excreted. As mentioned above, saturated fats are the main contributors to high blood cholesterol, or high LDL-cholesterol.

To reduce levels of blood cholesterol in general, you need to cut saturated fats from your diet and to increase the amount of exercise you do. Exercise can increase the levels of HDL-cholesterol, so that LDL-cholesterol can be carried away.

WHICH FATS ARE BAD?

Most people are aware that fats contribute to causing cancer, heart disease, obesity and weight gain. However, many people are confused by the popular knowledge that certain fats are good, while others are bad. If you remember only one fact from this chapter, it should be that all fats are equal when looking at the calorie contribution to the diet and the contribution to body fat.

When considering your general health and the prevention of lifestyle-related diseases, it is a good idea to reduce the saturated fat content of your diet and opt for more unsaturated fat sources (mono- or poly-unsaturated fats). When considering weight or fat loss, you need to take into consideration the total fat content of your diet, although new research shows that the body more easily burns up polyunsaturated fats than monounsaturated or saturated fats.

COMPARING FATS AND CARBOHYDRATES

Fats are packed with calories. For every 1 g of fat you consume, you receive 9 Calories of energy, whereas 1 g of carbohydrates or starches (such as bread, pasta, rice, etc.) or fruit provides only 4 Calories of energy. It can therefore be seen that fats provide more than double the amount of energy that carbohydrates do. In addition, while the body burns up any excess energy provided by starches or carbohydrates, it generally prefers to store any excess energy which is supplied by fats.

1 g OF MACRONUTRIENTS	CALORIES	kJ
Fat	9	37
Carbohydrate	4	17
Protein	4	17
Fruit	4	17
Alcohol	7	29
• 1 Calorie = 4.136 kJ		

Fat adds palatability to food, but provides the least satiety (feeling of fullness) of all the macronutients (carbohydrates, fats and proteins). However, the consumption of fats will delay the onset of feelings of hunger, so that more time will elapse before the next meal is needed. (Simply put, fats provide satiety *between* meals, while carbohydrates provide satiety *during* a meal.) Therefore, if you eat a meal that is low in fat or even fat free, it is normal for you to feel hungry again much sooner than if you ate a meal high in fat. Satiety during the meal is dependent on your carbohydrate intake, which means that you will not feel satisfied with that meal until you have consumed sufficient carbohydrates.

Recent studies have shown that if you overeat in terms of carbohydrates, your body will respond by increasing the rate at which it burns up carbohydrates. However the same does not always apply to fat. Overeating fats will therefore result in increased fat storage and therefore possible weight gain. This regulation of matching fat intake with fat burning is particularly poorly controlled in people with a tendency to obesity, but there also seems to be a variability between individuals. Also, if you overeat carbohydrates today, the body will automatically signal you to eat fewer carbohydrates the next day. Once again, the same internal regulation does not apply to fats. This is because the storage capacity of carbohydrate is very small, while the storage capacity of fats is huge. It may be said that the body notices when carbohydrates are taken in, while fat slips in unnoticed.

Some new scientific theories presently being tested show that some people may be better fat burners than others (and therefore less likely to gain weight if eating a high-fat diet) while others are better carbohydrate burners (and will therefore only maintain their weight as long as they stick to low-fat, high-carbohydrate diets). At the moment, this can only be determined individually in a laboratory using complicated and expensive testing methods, and further research is still needed.

FAT AND WEIGHT LOSS

Fat fulfils many important functions in the body, such as providing important vitamins and essential fatty acids, protecting the organs and nerves, providing insulation, allowing for storage of energy, etc. It is not a good idea, therefore, to remove all fat from your diet. This may also not be possible, as many fats are either unavoidable or hidden in your regular, everyday diet. It is a good idea, though, to make an effort to cut out fat wherever it is in your power to do so. Remember, also, that hidden fats are usually of the unhealthy, saturated, kind.

If you are eating at a restaurant, ordering your fish grilled rather than fried is a health-conscious choice. However, very few restaurants actually prepare their food *under a grill* as one would at home – usually the food is cooked *on a grill*, using a fair amount of fat. Even vegetables served in restaurants are often covered in butter or sauces. When, for example, you visit friends for coffee, you may resist the chocolate cake and choose a healthier bran muffin instead. Bear in mind, though, that the muffin still contains a notable amount of fat and that the coffee will probably be served with full-cream milk.

To sum up, therefore, it is a good idea to try to cut out the visible and hidden fats in your diet wherever possible and, when consciously adding fat to your diet, to make sure it is of the unsaturated kind.

CARBOHYDRATES AND WEIGHT LOSS

At this point you may ask why a virtually fat-free product like bread cannot be eaten in excess, if the body only stores fat and burns up carbohydrate. Here we need to consider the so-called energy balance theory:

energy consumed = energy spent $\rightarrow$ weight maintenance

This means that there needs to be a balance between the number of calories taken in by your body and the amount of energy you expend. The simple fact is that if more calories are taken in – from whatever source –

than can be expended, then the body may store some of the excess. More importantly, however, the body will not have to turn to its fat stores for fuel, and weight loss will not occur.

Drastically limiting your calorie intake does not provide the answer either. Fad diets involving milkshakes, pills, herbal remedies, limited types of foods, special food combinations and the like may allow you to lose weight rapidly in the initial stages. What is being lost, however, is often mostly weight in the form of muscle and water. This kind of fad diet may result in only a small amount of actual fat loss, and whatever weight loss you achieve will certainly not be permanent. Your body will identify the shortage of calories as a 'starvation state', and respond by lowering your metabolic rate and becoming more conservative about expending energy. Your body will actively try to conserve energy to protect itself.

So, the same person going for a run before starting a fad diet may, in fact, burn more calories than he or she would when going for the same run after having been on a starvation or fad diet for six weeks. Many people who have tried fad diets for any period of time will able to attest to the fact that weight loss slows markedly and may eventually stop altogether.

You will often hear people claiming to have either a slow or a fast metabolism. But what exactly is involved in the process of metabolism? Simply put, it may be said that your metabolism is basically your 'internal fire' that works just like the fire in the engine of a steam train. Your metabolism drives all the processes in your body – from digesting your food to making your muscles contract and relax when you exercise. If you stop adding fresh wood or coal to the fire, it will burn less fiercely and begin to form coals, and it may even die out eventually. The same principle applies to your body's metabolism – glucose (from carbo-hydrates) being the body's main energy fuel.

Most people who come and consult me find that they have slowed their metabolisms down to glowing coals rather than having built roaring fires. This is usually the result of years of fad diets, weight cycling, inactive lifestyles and unbalanced diets. And we all know that, when you add fresh wood to coals, the wood usually just smoulders, and does not actually start burning. Someone with a low metabolism will tell you that they almost feel the inches being added to their thighs or stomach when they eat a piece of cake.

What is needed is the rebuilding of a roaring fire so that, no matter what is fed into the fire, the body's metabolism just burns it all up. The only way to do this is to follow a high-carbohydrate, low-fat diet in conjunction with a regular program of exercise. I admit, it would be wonderful if grapefruit, chromium picolinate, kelp or ginseng worked a magical cure, but extensive studies have been done on all these substances. Nothing has been found to have a permanent effect, with the exception of exercise in combination with a balanced, high-carbohydrate, low-fat diet.

Remember that if you lose more than 1 kg per week, this usually means that you are also losing muscle and water, not just fat. A fat loss of 0.5–1 kg per week is realistic, attainable and maintainable.

MAINTAINING WEIGHT LOSS

Everyone who battles to lose weight will, sooner or later, ask the same burning question: how can weight loss be maintained permanently? In my experience, the answer to this question is probably one of the most sought-after pieces of information in the world. In fact, I have been told that statistics show that you have a greater chance of recovering from cancer than of losing weight and maintaining that weight loss for the rest of your life. Most people have, at some point in their lives, lost weight successfully. But how many of them have managed to maintain that weight loss ten years or even one year later? In the course of the last five years I have worked with hundreds of people trying to lose weight, and I have developed a weight-maintenance concept which works for most of my clients. I call it the 75%–25% concept.

What this means is the following: to maintain your weight loss, you must follow a low-fat lifestyle 75% of the time; 25% of the time you may relax your focus and eat what you like. It is important to note that this concept only works for weight maintenance and *not* for weight loss. Some people incorporate the 75%–25% concept into their lifestyles by following the low-fat lifestyle during the week and being less vigilant over weekends. Others stick to low-fat living when they are at home, but relax when they eat out. You may need to experiment and find what works best for you and your individual lifestyle.

Let me reiterate that diet alone does not do the trick. Scientific research has shown that the most successful way to maintain long-term weight loss is *dietary control in combination with a moderate exercise program.*

WHAT SHOULD I BE EATING IF I WANT TO LOSE WEIGHT?

A low-fat diet consisting of mostly carbohydrates, fruit and vegetables, and moderate amounts of protein and dairy, is recommended for weight loss and weight maintenance. The guidelines set out in this book should be adequate to help you design your own eating plan. However, if you would like a diet carefully tailored to your own specific needs, I recommend that you consult a registered dietician. (Refer to the useful contact numbers given at the back of the book.) There are many people who call themselves nutritionists or dieticians while not being properly qualified. All dieticians have spent a minimum of four years studying at a university. An easy way to find out if someone is registered or not, is to ask whether medical aid claims can be made – only registered dieticians can be contracted into medical aids.

A varied, balanced diet is demonstrated in the following diagram of a food pyramid.

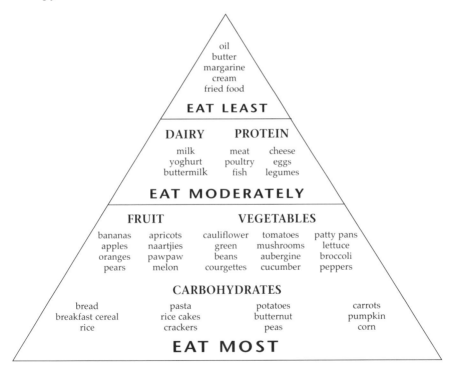

GUIDELINES FOR A BALANCED, DAILY EATING PLAN FOR WEIGHT LOSS

It is important that you follow a varied, balanced daily diet, including some food from each of the following food groups: carbohydrates, fruit, vegetables, protein, milk or dairy products and fat. Below I have outlined the recommended portions.

Carbohydrates

6–10 portions per day (spread over the day) where the lower amounts are for women not physically active and the upper spectrum is for physically active men (these amounts may not be relevant for children or athletes or other groups with special requirements).

1 portion = 1 slice bread *or* 3 Pro-Vita biscuits *or* 1 Weet-bix *or* ½ cup cooked rice or pasta *or* 1 medium potato

Fruit

3–5 portions per day based on the same criteria as for carbohydrates

1 portion = 1 banana *or* 1 pear *or* 2 naartjies *or* 1 orange *or* 2 plums *or* 1 apple *or* 1 tbsp raisins *or* 4 dried apricot halves *or* 2 prunes *or* half a glass of fruit juice

'Free' vegetables

At least three different kinds of vegetables per day, eaten freely and used as gap-fillers

Free vegetables = asparagus, artichokes, broccoli, cauliflower, celery, Brussels sprouts, cabbage, spinach, lettuce, cucumber (fresh or pickled), peppers, radish, spring onions, tomato, aubergine, marrows, patty pans, green beans, gems, mushrooms

'Carbohydrate' vegetables

The following vegetables are not regarded as 'free' vegetables, but counted as carbohydrate portions.

1 portion = 1 cup carrots *or* 1 cup butternut *or* 1 cup peas *or* 1 cup pumpkin *or* 1 cup beetroot *or* 1 medium potato

Protein
4–6 portions per day based on the same criteria as for carbohydrates
   1 portion =   1 matchbox-sized piece of chicken, cheese or lean red meat *or* 2 matchbox-sized pieces of white fish or cottage cheese

Milk or dairy products
2–3 portions per day, where two is sufficient for men and three is necessary for women and children
   1 portion =   1 cup fat-free/skim milk *or* 1 small tub (175 ml) fat-free fruit yoghurt/plain yoghurt

Fat
0–3 portions per day depending on whether any hidden fats have been consumed that day (note that unsaturated sources of fat are recommended)
   1 portion =   1 tsp oil or margarine *or* 2 tsp low-fat margarine *or* 2 tsp low-fat mayonnaise or salad cream *or* 2 tsp peanut butter *or* ¼ avocado *or* 4 cashew nuts

THE SPECIFICS
OF A HEALTHY DAILY EATING PLAN

Below I have set out an ideal eating plan for a forty-year-old woman who does 30–45 minutes of exercise 3–4 times per week and who needs to lose weight.

BREAKFAST
- ❖ 2 slices whole-wheat toast with thinly spread jam or fat-free cottage cheese or fishpaste or Marmite or mashed banana (use Flora extra light margarine if necessary)
  or 1½ cups All-Bran flakes *or* 2 Weet-bix with fat-free milk/yoghurt
  or ⅔ cup low-fat muesli *or* 1 packet Oatso Easy
- ❖ do not consume more than 3 eggs per week
- ❖ 1 bowl of fruit salad

MID-MORNING SNACK
- ❖ 1 piece of fruit
- ❖ 1 small tub (175 ml) fat-free fruit yoghurt or fat-free plain yoghurt

LUNCH

❖ 2 slices bread *or* 4 Ryvitas *or* a large baked potato with fat-free cottage cheese or fat-free cream cheese *or* 2 low-fat cheese wedges *or* 1 slice turkey or smoked chicken *or* ½ can tuna in brine *or* ¼ avocado

❖ Use mustard, chutney or 2 tsp Trim mayonnaise (Knorr oil-free Thousand Island dressing mixed with fat-free plain yoghurt makes a tasty mayonnaise)

❖ Salads with balsamic vinegar or other fat-free dressings *or* a bowl of free vegetable soup (see pages 86 and 88 for 'free' soup recipes, or make your own soup using the 'free' vegetables listed on page 18)

AFTERNOON SNACK

❖ 3 Pro-Vita biscuits with Marmite or fat-free cottage cheese or 2 tsp peanut butter
or 1 small bran muffin
and 1 SAD fruit bar
and 1 low-fat Cup-a-Soup

SUPPER

❖ A cooked meal with 3 matchbox-sized pieces (90 g) of fish or chicken or lean red meat (try not to eat red meat more than three times per week, as it is high in saturated fats)

❖ Fill up on lots of free vegetables and salads and a large baked potato, *or* 1 cup of cooked rice or pasta (put a dollop of fat-free cottage or cream cheese in your potato instead of butter).

❖ Use no oil or other fat when cooking – use chutney, wine, tomato or soy sauce, stock cubes, soup powder and water for browning, thickening and stir-frying.

EVENING SNACK

❖ 1 small tub (175 ml) fat-free yoghurt
or 1 cup Milo made with fat-free milk and 1 heaped tsp Milo powder

OTHER

Drink no more than four cups of tea or coffee per day using fat-free milk and substituting sugar with sweeteners if you use two or more teaspoons of sugar per cup. Herbal tea can be used freely if desired.

WHAT ABOUT ALCOHOL?

Whether alcohol is allowed or not is surely one of the most common questions I am asked when discussing a low-fat diet with a client. Most people are surprised to learn that alcohol contains no fat and is therefore essentially a fat-free product. Alcohol is high in calories, however, and it may also interfere with your body's normal metabolism. If you are trying to lose weight, I recommend that you moderate your alcohol intake.

One of the main reasons why many beer-drinkers are overweight, is because of the high-fat or high-calorie foods they consume while drinking beer, for example potato chips, biltong or peanuts, to name but a few. When you are having a drink, it is also important to note which mixers you may be using, for example Coke, lemonade, orange juice etc. Each additional mixer adds to the number of calories you are consuming. Lastly, remember that alcohol increases your appetite, as well as relaxing you and making you less careful. You may, therefore, be more easily tempted by high-fat or high-calorie foods.

The prudent (healthy) guidelines recommend no more than 2 alcoholic beverages a day for women and 3 for men. This is not a sexist arrangement, but due to the fact that men have more of the alcohol-detoxifying enzyme than women do.

1 alcoholic beverage   =   125 ml white or red wine *or* 1 tot spirits
or half a beer *or* half a cider

Generally, I encourage my clients who want to lose weight to substitute all or some of their supper carbohydrates if they are planning to indulge in 2–3 alcoholic beverages. Alcohol adds extra calories to your energy intake, and this needs to be taken into account. So, for instance, if you are following the guidelines set out above and want to have two glasses of wine with your supper, then you could leave out the potato, pasta or rice and just have chicken or fish with salad and lots of 'free' vegetables.

WILL IT HELP ME LOSE WEIGHT IF I DRINK PLENTY OF WATER?

Contrary to popular belief, drinking a lot of water will not help you lose weight faster, but it will help fill you up and make you feel less hungry. The most important reasons for drinking water, however, are probably that it helps prevent constipation and dehydration, and that it keeps your body flushed of toxins and other waste products. Try to drink 6–8 glasses of water per day (in winter hot water with a slice of lemon, some ginger or a sprig of mint is pleasant). Also, when you find yourself feeling hungry, ask yourself whether you may not be thirsty rather than hungry. I have come across numerous clients who actually confuse hunger with thirst, and eat in an attempt to satisfy their thirst.

THE ROLE OF EXERCISE IN LOSING OR MAINTAINING WEIGHT

Although the main concern of this book is to describe how to decrease your total dietary caloric intake by cutting out the fats, it would be incomplete if no mention was made of the role of exercise. When it comes to weight control, exercise is just as important as diet. Just how this works can be explained by referring to the energy balance theory, as discussed before (*see* p. 14). The relevant principle implies that if you want to maintain your weight, then the amount of energy you take in through your diet must equal the amount of energy you expend in the course of your daily activities. If you want to lose weight, therefore, the energy you take in through your diet must be less than the energy you expend. If your aim is weight loss, the best results are achieved by simultaneouly reducing your energy intake and increasing your energy output by exercising.

If you merely reduce your daily calorie intake, you may activate your body's survival response, which means that your metabolism will start slowing down (*see also* p. 15). Exercise can help to prevent this by maintaining your metabolic rate, and even increasing it. The more muscle you have, the more calories are burnt up, so it is definitely worth developing and toning your muscles by exercising.

The safest, most easily measurable and controllable way of increasing your daily activity levels is to start a formal exercise program. Depending on your personal needs, this can take place in a gym, in the nearest park, as part of a running or walking club, in your own home, or wherever. Most of my clients find that it is necessary to formalize and plan an exercise regime so that it becomes a priority in their lives. If you do not currently follow a formal exercise program, I recommend that you choose a form of exercise that you really enjoy, and start off slowly.

Although I have been running my practice in a gym and health club environment for the past five years, I do not have the skills to prescribe specialized exercise programs. I strongly believe in referring my clients to professionals who are properly qualified to prescribe exercise, for example biokineticists, sports scientists, physiotherapists and personal trainers. These trained experts will help you design a program that provides variety, and that allows you to safely adjust the intensity and the frequency when necessary. Stick to your routine, and you will find it becoming an invaluable lifelong habit.

Having mentioned that you should choose a form of exercise that you enjoy, I would like to add a very important point for you to bear in mind. In my experience, some people start an exercise program and love it passionately almost from the start. Others will always find exercising a bothersome chore, no matter what they try. However, even reluctant exercisers often admit that, while they may feel very negative at the start of their daily exercise, they feel really good afterwards. Once you have completed your gym session, swim or brisk walk, you may even feel great. The reason is that exercise triggers your body to release endorphins, the so-called 'feel-good' hormones.

In addition to making you feel good, exercise has been shown to have many other benefits. A vast and rapidly growing body of research is proving that exercise can assist in preventing cancer, lowering blood cholesterol levels, lowering blood pressure, easing control of diabetes and preventing osteoporosis, to name but a few serious conditions.

Exercise does not have to be limited to a formal training program, however. If you decide to change your eating habits, why not change some of your other habits as well? Make a point of always using the stairs instead of the lift, for instance. Rather than circling the car park endlessly waiting for a vacant spot near the entrance of the building, park your car where you find space and then make the most of your short walk. (Personally, I am constantly amused by the many gym-goers who fight over the parking bays close to the gym entrance so that they do not have too far to walk and yet, once inside, they may run and cycle many kilometers on the machines.)

Many people become discouraged about exercising, because they have been told that it is necessary to exercise for an hour or more if they want to burn fat. The reality of the situation is that most people do not, in fact, have the time or patience to exercise for 1–2 hours 3–5 times per week. It is far more realistic and practical to set yourself a goal of exercising for

30–45 minutes 3–5 times per week. Exercising at a high intensity for a shorter period of time actually results in more fat from your fat stores being utilized in the hours following the exercise in order to replenish the energy stores in your muscles.

To sum up, I recommend that you seek professional advice before embarking on any exercise program. And remember – choose an exercise that you really enjoy, as you will need to continue exercising for the rest of your life, even once your goal weight has been achieved.

MIND OVER FOOD – LEARNING TO LIVE WITH LOW FAT

THE HARD PART IS MAKING UP YOUR MIND TO DO SOMETHING; THE EASY PART IS STICKING TO IT

PAT'S STORY

Once my friends started seeing the great changes in me, they all asked if it was difficult for me to follow the low-fat lifestyle. I told them that – once I had made up my mind to follow the low-fat lifestyle – it was easy. Perhaps what made it easier was the fact that I had had four small strokes and this made me realize how important diet is. After returning to the UK, I was having Christmas lunch with some ladies from my health club there and they asked me the secret of my obvious success. I told them briefly what I had done, mainly just cut out all the fats. The replies going round the table of ten were, 'I like my butter', 'I love my beef', 'I can't cook without olive oil', etc. Finally, in exasperation, I stood up and said 'OK, then stay fat!'

SUCCESS DEPENDS ON YOUR COMMITMENT AND MOTIVATION

For Peta, the key to success was the realization that no dietician could give her a miracle drug, food, substance or even food combination that would help her lose weight and maintain that weight loss. From the very beginning she realized that she would have to take responsibility for her own actions and that her success would depend on her commitment and motivation to stick to the low-fat lifestyle and exercise plan. It was this realization that helped her lose a large amount of weight and then maintain that weight loss a year later while still enjoying a normal, healthy life.

EAT TO LOSE

Deidre found it miraculous that she did not have to starve and deprive herself to lose weight – she could still eat lots of normal, everyday food-stuffs. One of the most rewarding things for me, as her dietician, is Deidre's genuine surprise when she stands on the scale every couple of weeks and she has either lost weight or maintained her weight (despite holidays, celebrations, and so forth). Most people seem to believe in the saying 'no pain, no gain'– also when it comes to losing weight. Deidre still cannot quite believe that you can eat plenty of tasty food, and yet lose weight.

YOU DO NOT HAVE TO KEEP TO THE
LOW-FAT LIFESTYLE PLAN ALL THE TIME

One of the things that discourages people from starting a 'diet' or an eating plan to lose weight, is their concern that they may have to stick to the eating plan for the rest of their lives if they want to maintain their weight loss. Quite correctly, weight maintenance is an important concern. Patsy followed the low-fat plan and reached her goal weight. She has also now been maintaining her weight for several months. All she is doing is eating according to the maintenance concept mentioned earlier (*see* p. 16). She follows the low-fat lifestyle plan during the week, and eats what she likes over weekends. Come Christmas, Easter or long weekends, she continues to maintain her new weight.

DON'T GO HUNGRY – YOU ARE ONLY HUMAN AND
ARE SURE TO SLIP UP IF YOU ARE HUNGRY,
SO BE KIND TO YOURSELF.

Janine loves the fact that she is never hungry – this is indeed another one of the secrets to success. Before going to a cocktail party or to a dinner party where you will be eating rather late, for instance, 'fill up' at home with soup, salad, fruit or yoghurt. You will then be able to resist the pre-dinner offers of chips and dips, sausage rolls, samoosas and other snacks.

ACKNOWLEDGE WHY YOU EAT

Many of the people who consult me are 'emotional eaters'. One client told me that she always asks herself, as she is about to take a bite of chocolate, for example, why she is doing it. If she is eating just for the taste, she has one bite and puts the rest away. If she is hungry, she first makes herself a sandwich and, invariably, after eating the sandwich she no longer feels like eating the chocolate. If she is bored, stressed, depressed or tired – all of which can explain why people overindulge – she does something else to address her feelings. She may rest, exercise, go for a massage or even scream and shout at the barking dog next door.

REALIZE THAT WE ARE ALL IN THE SAME BOAT

My clients find it very motivating to realize that, after a certain age, most people – including dieticians(!) – have no choice but to follow a low-fat lifestyle and a regular exercise plan if they want to remain healthy and energized. Weight loss and/or weight maintenance become bonuses – the real aim of the low-fat lifestyle is improved general health, with the additional benefits of disease prevention (especially relating to cancer, heart disease, diabetes and high blood pressure).

MAKE HABIT-CHANGING YOUR SHORT-TERM GOAL AND WEIGHT LOSS YOUR LONG-TERM GOAL

During the first six weeks of following your low-fat lifestyle plan, your main aim should be to learn to identify bad habits and to change them. This relates to how and where you do your shopping, what you choose to buy, which methods you use to prepare and cook your food, when and why you eat, and so forth. If you are an ex yo-yo dieter, repeatedly having lost weight only to gain it all again, it often takes up to six weeks for your body to adapt to the changes in your diet and to start burning fat.

Though weight loss may not occur immediately, there are a number of other positive changes that will soon be evident. You may experience improved mood, improved energy levels, fewer cravings, better control of blood sugar levels, improved sleeping habits, improved bowel habits, improved ability to deal with stress, etc. If you want to check your general progress in terms of burning fat, use more reliable measurements of progress than your bathroom scale. You may find that you gain a little weight initially, as exercise often increases heavy muscle gain fairly rapidly early on. The waistband of your trousers may be a better guide to how your shape is changing.

RESIST TELLING PEOPLE THAT YOU ARE
TRYING TO LOSE WEIGHT

When you are with friends, never give losing weight as the reason for turning down a second helping or dessert, for instance. If you do, you can be guaranteed that your host and fellow diners will all collaborate in telling you that you do not need to lose weight. The fact that you are abstaining may make them feel guilty, because they may realize that they should be doing the same. They may even subtly pressure you, because if you do give in, they will feel better about their own indulgence. If you say that you have an upset stomach, however, or that you need to watch your cholesterol intake, people are likely to be far more understanding.

SET YOURSELF SHORT-TERM, EASILY ATTAINABLE GOALS

Realistically speaking, the average weight loss you can expect per week is approximately 0.5–1 kg. If your goal is to lose 15 kg, try not to look at the whole five months that you will probably need in which to lose that weight. Fix your focus on the first four weeks, and concentrate on losing 3 kg. Once you have achieved that goal, you will be proud and motivated and have the courage to focus on the next four weeks and the next 3 kg.

ACCEPT THAT WEIGHT LOSS IS NOT EASY

At the very beginning of your new eating and exercise plan, accept the fact that there is no easy way out – weight loss is not easy. If you are looking for an easy solution, then a fad diet is what you will find. Fad diets usually result in easy water and muscle loss, and an immediate weight gain when you begin eating normally again. Interestingly, I find that some of my most successful clients are those who have tried all the 'easy' methods over the years and, through much anguish and financial loss, have finally come to realize and accept that *there is no easy way.*

In my own practice I often use a 12-week weight management program to get my clients started on their new low-fat lifestyle. To put the program in perspective, I ask them: 'How about spending a period of 12 weeks out of 52 weeks of a year in your life working really hard at something to achieve that goal that you so badly want?' I remind them of how long it took them to gain the weight they want to lose, and point out that it is unrealistic to expect to lose that weight in a shorter time.

CHAPTER TWO

Shopping Guide

UNDERSTANDING FOOD LABELS

As consumers gain more knowledge and become more aware of the fat content of what they are eating, they need to be able to obtain nutritional information from food labels in order to make informed choices. Food labels can provide a wealth of useful information, but it is essential to understand and use the information on food labels correctly.

Ingredients are listed in order of weight. They help you make comparisons between similar products, to establish value for money and to avoid ingredients that you do not eat. Therefore, if fat in any form appears high up on the list, then there is a good chance that it may be a high-fat product.

LOW-OIL SALAD DRESSING

INGREDIENTS: Water, vinegar, sunflower oil (10.5%), modified maize starch, sucrose, mustard flour, sodium chloride, lemon juice, citric acid, sodium saccharin (0.02%), spices, stabilisers, emulsifiers, colourant. Preserved with potassium sorbate.

NUTRITIONAL INFORMATION

TYPICAL VALUES	per 100g	per tablespoon (15 ml)
Energy	618 kJ	97 kJ
Protein	0.8 g	0.1 g
Carbohydrate	11.9 g	1.8 g
(Sugars)	(5.2 g)	(0.8 g)
Fat	10.4 g	1.6 g
(Saturated)	(1.9 g	(0.2 g)
Fibre	trace	trace
Sodium	900 mg	100 mg

A claim such as 'low-oil' must be backed up by stating the exact amounts in the nutritional information breakdown.

Manufacturers cannot make statements such as 'low-oil' unless the products contains no more than 75% of the oil of a similar product about which no claim is made. In other words, if a product normally has 10 g of fat and an equivalent low-fat product is brought out, it only needs to have 7 g of fat to be called a low-fat product. In fact, the above product should be called a 'reduced-fat' product, as low-fat products should have less than 3 g of fat per 100 g.

The law prohibits certain claims being made on food labels:

❖ No label may claim that a food product possesses health-giving properties.

❖ A label may not claim that a product is free of a substance like cholesterol, for instance, if all the other products in the same category are also free of that substance, for example all margarines and oils are cholesterol free.

As consumers we should all be proactively looking for a label, reading the nutritional information on that label and using this knowledge to inform our product choice. If it is true that we are what we eat, good labelling will allow us to make informed choices in moving towards better health through sensible eating practices.

Unfortunately, it is very difficult to legislate in terms of labelling on imported foodstuffs – so keep your wits about you when you are trying to assess these products.

How to assess fat content

❖ When you read the ingredient list on the label, look to see whether fat is listed as one of the 'Top Three' ingredients. The ingredients present in a product are listed in descending order, so this means that if fat appears high up on the list, the particular foodstuff probably has a high fat content.

❖ If fat is listed several times as an ingredient and given various names (hidden under the following 'aliases': hydrogenated fat, vegetable fat, vegetable oil, animal fat, shortening, lard, cream, butter, margarine), then the foodstuff is probably high in fat.

❖ Look for the fat content of the food by weight to work out how many grams of fat a typical serving or portion of this food will add to your total daily fat intake. (Use < 5 g per portion as a guideline.)

❖ Remember that the terms 'low-fat' or 'reduced fat' do not mean that a product is 'fat free'!

SHOPPING LISTS

The shopping lists given in this chapter have highlighted *low-fat foods per portion* only. No foodstuffs have been considered for other components such as fibre, trans fatty acids, preservatives or salt. However, it is safe to say that the quantities of all the substances used by food manufacturers are safe and controlled by legislation and that, when consumed in moderate amounts as part of a balanced diet, they should cause no harm. This may exclude persons with specific medical problems or special dietary needs. If you are unsure whether or not a food is suitable, it is a good idea to seek advice from a registered dietitian.

Labels on food products generally display nutritional information per 100 g. This information is often not immediately useful to the consumer, because one does not necessarily eat only 100 g of a particular foodstuff. For example, it is unlikely that anyone will consume 100 g of salad dressing all at once or, similarly, that anyone will eat only 100 g of a 350-g serving of a ready-made convenience meal. It is also difficult to convert 100 g of a foodstuff into an easily measurable household portion. The following lists have been compiled with this in mind, and they therefore indicate the fat content of foods per portion size rather than per 100 g.

Where portion sizes have not been provided by manufacturers, these have been estimated using reliable, commonly used dietetic tools. Where portion sizes are not applicable, for example for coatings and flavourings, these have been omitted.

As a general guideline, only foods containing 5 g of fat or less per portion have been included. Products not included in this list may have been omitted either due to a lack of nutritional information provided or because they cannot be considered low-fat products by the authors.

In compiling this list, no single manufacturer has been targeted or given special consideration, and none has paid for advertising space. The information provided in this shopping list can be obtained by any consumer – we have simply done that for you to make your shopping easier. The list is merely a guide to what is available and it should be used with caution. All the relevant information was correct and up to date at the time of printing. As new products constantly appear on the market, though, it is understandable that, by the time this book reaches consumers, there will be new and suitable products available which are not listed here.

BREAKFAST CEREALS AND PORRIDGES

PRODUCT NAME	PORTION SIZE	FAT CONTENT (per serving)
Cereals		
ALPEN		
Original Swiss Muesli	3 tbsp	2.70 g
Tropical Muesli	3 tbsp	2.80 g
BOKOMO		
Bran Flakes	1 heaped cup	0.90 g
Bran-Bix	2 biscuits	3.30 g
Corn Flakes	1 heaped cup	0.10 g
Frosted Crunchies	1 heaped cup	0.20 g
Fruity Flakes	1 heaped cup	1.00 g
Fruity-Bix	2 biscuits	1.00 g
Honey Flakes	1 heaped cup	0.50 g
Mabel's Fruit Munch	½ cup	4.83 g
Morning Harvest Muesli	½ cup	2.20 g
Muesli Raisin	½ cup	4.20 g
Nu-Bix	2 biscuits	2.80 g
Oat-Bix	2 biscuits	1.20 g
Puffed Wheat	1 heaped cup	0.30 g
Rainbow Crunchies	1 heaped cup	0.20 g
Strawberry Crunchies	1 heaped cup	0.20 g
Weet-Bix	2 biscuits	0.80 g
Wheat Flakes	1 heaped cup	0.80 g
HARVELD		
New Day Muesli	½ cup	1.53 g
KELLOGGS		
All-Bran Flakes	1 heaped cup	1.02 g
Choco Krispies	1 heaped cup	0.08 g
Chocos	1 heaped cup	0.40 g
Corn Flakes	1 heaped cup	0.26 g
Corn Pops	1 heaped cup	0.50 g
Crunchy Nut Corn Flakes	1 heaped cup	0.90 g
Froot Loops	1 heaped cup	0.50 g
Frosties	1 heaped cup	0.05 g
Fruitful All-Bran Flakes	1 cup	1.60 g
Hi-Fibre Bran	5 tbsp	1.60 g
Honey O's	1 heaped cup	1.20 g
Just Right	1 heaped cup	0.30 g

PRODUCT NAME	PORTION SIZE	FAT CONTENT (per serving)
Low-Fat Toasted Muesli	3 tbsp	1.70 g
Nutrific	2 biscuits	0.80 g
Rice Krispies	1 heaped cup	0.30 g
Special K	1 heaped cup	0.33 g
Strawberry Pops	1 heaped cup	0.08 g
NATURE'S SOURCE		
Choc Bitz	½ cup	4.80 g
Ideal Mix Muesli Crunch	½ cup	2.58 g
Ideal Mix Nutzy Crunch	½ cup	2.12 g
Ideal Mix Original	½ cup	1.62 g
Luxury Swiss Muesli	½ cup	1.53 g
Nut Feast	½ cup	2.50 g
Nutty-O's	¾ cup	4.86 g
Orange & Chocolate Cereal	½ cup	4.70 g
Strawberry & Yoghurt Cereal	½ cup	4.98 g
Toasted Nut Crunch	½ cup	3.21 g
Tropical Cluster	½ cup	2.84 g
Wafflers	1 heaped cup	1.00 g
NESTLÉ		
Junior Cereal	¾ cup	1.10 g
NATIONAL BRANDS		
ProNutro	5 heaped tbsp	3.80 g
ProNutro Flakes	3 heaped tbsp	0.70 g
Wholewheat ProNutro	5 heaped tbsp	2.90 g
PICK 'N PAY		
Corn Flakes	1 heaped cup	0.40 g
High Fibre Luxury Muesli	½ cup	1.30 g
No Name Brand Bran Flakes	1 heaped cup	0.90 g
Popped Rice	1 heaped cup	0.40 g
No Name Shredded Bran	1 heaped cup	0.80 g
Toasted Caramel Crunch	1 heaped cup	2.45 g
Wholewheat Malt Munchies	1 heaped cup	1.00 g
POST		
Grape-Nuts Flakes	1 cup	0.60 g
Shredded Wheat	1 biscuit	0.70 g
Shreddies	⅔ cup	0.60 g
SPAR		
Breakfast Crunch Toasted Muesli	½ cup	3.21 g
WEIGH-LESS		
High-Bulk Muesli	½ cup	1.50 g

PRODUCT NAME	PORTION SIZE	FAT CONTENT (per serving)
WOOLWORTHS		
Bran Flakes	1 heaped cup	0.00 g
Breakfast Bran	5 tbsp	1.23 g
Breakfast Muesli	½ cup	3.00 g
Corn Flakes	1 heaped cup	0.10 g
Crisped Rice	1 heaped cup	0.00 g
Crunchy Chocolate Clusters	½ cup	4.86 g
Crunchy Mixed Fruit Clusters	½ cup	4.62 g
Frosted Flakes	1 heaped cup	0.21 g
Fruit & Flake	1 heaped cup	1.65 g
Luxury Fruit & Nut Muesli	⅔ cup	3.10 g
Luxury Muesli	½ cup	2.30 g
Muesli Breakfast Biscuits	2 biscuits	2.20 g
Oat-o Nut	½ cup	4.90 g
Unsweetened Bran Muesli	⅔ cup	2.45 g
Wheat Breakfast Biscuits	2 biscuits	0.80 g
Wildberry Breakfast Biscuits	1 cup	0.70 g
VITAL		
High-Fibre Low-Cholesterol Muesli	½ cup	3.45 g

Porridges

BOKOMO		
Quick-Cooking Oats	4 heaped tbsp	2.60 g
HINDS		
Kreemy Meel	¼ cup	0.00 g
Maltabella	¼ cup	0.00 g
JUNGLE OATS CO.		
Jungle Oats	4 heaped tbsp	3.60 g
Oat Bran	4 heaped tbsp	3.40 g
Oatso Easy – Natural	1 sachet	3.10 g
Peaches & Cream	1 sachet	2.10 g
Raisin Bran Malt	1 sachet	3.90 g
Bananas & Cream / Strawberry Apple & Honey / Caramel	1 sachet	2.70 g
Taystee Maize	3 heaped tbsp	0.90 g
Taystee Wheat	3 heaped tbsp	0.60 g
Taystee Wheat Bran	3 heaped tbsp	0.80 g
PICK 'N PAY NO NAME BRAND		
One-minute Oats	4 heaped tbsp	2.60 g

PRODUCT NAME	PORTION SIZE	FAT CONTENT (per serving)
TIGER OATS CO.		
Oatmeal	4 heaped tbsp	2.60 g
WOOLWORTHS		
Oats	4 heaped tbsp	1.04 g

BAKERY

PRODUCT NAME	PORTION SIZE	FAT CONTENT (per serving)
Breads & Rolls		
ALBANY		
High Fibre Brown	2 slices	1.70 g
High Protein White	2 slices	1.60 g
Wholewheat Brown	2 slices	2.10 g
Slimslice		
Brown	3 slices	0.80 g
Stone-ground brown	3 slices	1.60 g
White	3 slices	0.50 g
BLUE RIBBON		
High Fibre	2 slices	0.67 g
Nutty Wheat	2 slices	1.11 g
White Toaster	2 slices	0.77 g
Wholegrain	2 slices	1.24 g
DUENS		
Brown	2 slices	1.11 g
Brown Dumpy	2 slices	1.70 g
High Fibre	2 slices	0.98 g
Purity Dumpy	2 slices	2.10 g
Super White	2 slices	1.96 g
Wheat Brown	2 slices	1.52 g
Wheat Brown Dumpy	2 slices	1.10 g
White Dumpy	2 slices	1.60 g
PICK 'N PAY FOODHALL		
Berliner Rye Bread	2 slices	0.00 g
Floured Baps	1 bap	1.00 g
Italian Bread & Roll Selection	2 slices/1 roll	0.35 g

PRODUCT NAME	PORTION SIZE	FAT CONTENT (per serving)
Italian Flatbreads		
Olive, Pimento & Garlic	¼ flatbread	3.3 g
Spring Onion & Parsley	¼ flatbread	3.3 g
Sun-dried Tomato & Parsley	¼ flatbread	3.3 g
Italian Olive Rolls	1 roll	4.28 g
White/Brown Pita Bread	1 pita	0.00 g
White/Brown Ready-to-Bake Rolls	1 roll	1.15 g
UNCLE SALIE'S		
Traditional Cape Homemade Brown	2 slices	1.95 g
WOOLWORTHS		
3 Korn Bread	1 slice	1.12 g
American Bagels	1 bagel	4.00 g
Brown Bread	2 slices	1.60 g
Brown Super Bread	2 slices	1.44 g
Floured Baps	1 bap	1.20 g
Fruited Seedloaf	2 slices	1.60 g
Hamburger; Hot dog; Soft Sesame	1 roll	2.40 g
Hamburger; Hot dog; Soft White Rolls	1 roll	1.80 g
Kitke Rolls	1 roll	2.50 g
Olive Italian Bread & Rolls	1 roll	1.95 g
Plain Italian Bread & Rolls	1 roll	1.30 g
Plain Seedloaf	2 slices	1.60 g
Portuguese Rolls	1 roll	1.20 g
Rye Bread	2 slices	0.75 g
Seeded Rolls	1 roll	2.40 g
Sliced Wholewheat Bread	2 slices	1.44 g
Sunflower Seed Rye Bread	2 slices	3.00 g
White Super Bread	2 slices	1.44 g
White Toaster Bread	2 thick slices	1.60 g
Wholegrain Super Bread	2 slices	1.60 g
Wholewheat Brown Bread	2 slices	1.60 g
Wholewheat Rye Bread	2 slices	1.50 g

Fresh Confectionery
GOLDEN CLOUD		
Cape-Style Bread Mix	2 slices	0.00 g
Pancake Mix	3 pancakes	1.50 g
MOIRS		
All-purpose Dough Mix Pizza Base	1 medium base	0.00 g

PRODUCT NAME	PORTION SIZE	FAT CONTENT (per serving)
PICK 'N PAY FOODHALL		
British Crumpets	2 crumpets	0.00 g
Sponge Cakes	1 small wedge	trace
Meringues		
Baskets/Mini baskets	each	0.00 g
Pavlova	⅛ pavlova	0.00 g
Rosettes	2 rosettes	0.00 g
PILLSBURY		
Banana Nut Loaf/Muffin Mix	2 slices or 1 muffin	4.80 g
Crumpet/Waffle Mix		
Raisin & Honey	3 x 10-cm crumpet or 1 waffle	1.10 g
Orange Blossom	3 x 10-cm crumpet or 1 waffle	1.20 g
Lemon Poppyseed	3 x 10-cm crumpet or 1 waffle	2.10 g
Chocolate Sprinkle	3 x 10-cm crumpet or 1 waffle	1.80 g
RECORD		
Pizza Base Mix	20-cm base	3.75 g
WHEATON'S		
Brumpets		
Choc Chip	3 crumpets	2.4 g
Other flavours	3 crumpets	3.3 g
WOOLWORTHS		
Crumpets	2 crumpets	0.00 g
English Muffins	2 muffins	0.50 g

Frozen Confectionery

PRODUCT NAME	PORTION SIZE	FAT CONTENT (per serving)
ITAL PIZZA		
Pizza Bases	25-cm base	0.84 g
JULIES		
Garlic or Herb Foccacia	25-cm base	1.80 g
PICK 'N PAY CHOICE		
Phyllo Pastry	N/A	trace
Pizza Bases	25-cm base	trace
WEIGH-LESS		
Bran Muffin Dough	2 small muffins	0.34 g

PRODUCT NAME	PORTION SIZE	FAT CONTENT (per serving)
Biscuits & Rusks		
BAKERS		
Boudoir	3 biscuits	1.11 g
Ginger Nuts	3 biscuits	2.61 g
Italian Wafers		
Chocolate	3 wafers	3.05 g
Butterscotch	3 wafers	3.64 g
Strawberry	3 wafers	3.34 g
Marie	3 biscuits	1.80 g
Tennis	3 biscuits	4.80 g
BAUMANN'S		
Marie	3 biscuits	1.80 g
Match	3 biscuits	4.20 g
Tennis	3 biscuits	4.68 g
BOKOMO		
Rusks		
Buttermilk	1 rusk	4.02 g
Plain	2 rusks	4.32 g
Wholewheat; Muesli	1 rusk	4.20 g
NOLA		
Ouma Rusks		
Aniseed	1 rusk	4.86 g
Buttermilk	1 rusk	4.67 g
Condensed Milk	1 rusk	4.71 g
Muesli	1 rusk	4.79 g
Wholewheat	1 rusk	4.98 g
PICK 'N PAY NO NAME BRAND		
Marie	3 biscuits	2.0 g
Sliced Buttermilk Rusks	2 rusks	2.16 g
Tennis	3 biscuits	4.40 g
WOOLWORTHS		
Italian Biscotti	3 slices	2.60 g
Crackers		
BAKALI'S		
Rice Cakes	2 slices	0.50 g
BAKERS		
Bacon Kips	3 biscuits	3.17 g
Cheddars	3 biscuits	2.10 g
Cream Crackers	3 crackers	2.70 g

PRODUCT NAME	PORTION SIZE	FAT CONTENT (per serving)
Pro-Vita	3 slices	1.40 g
Salt & Vinegar Kips	3 biscuits	3.17 g
Spring Onion Kips	3 biscuits	3.17 g
Tomato Kips	3 biscuits	3.17 g
BAUMANN'S		
Habits	3 biscuits	1.50 g
CARR'S		
Water Biscuit	3 biscuits	0.90 g
FINN CRISP		
Dark Caraway	3 slices	0.00 g
Hi-Fibre Crispbread		
Harvest Wheat	2 slices	1.88 g
Original Rye	2 slices	0.65 g
Sourdough	3 slices	0.00 g
MOZMARKS		
Matzos	1 large sheet	trace
NABISCO		
Crackermate Lites	3 biscuits	1.50g
PICK 'N PAY CHOICE		
Italian Classic Breadsticks	3 sticks	1.63 g
Italian Classic Toasts	2 slices	0.96 g
PYOTT'S		
Cheddanuts	15 biscuits	4.12 g
Cheese Snaps	15 biscuits	3.28 g
Cream Crackers	3 biscuits	3.64 g
Hi Toast Crackerbread		
Original	3 slices	0.15 g
Pepper & Herb	3 slices	0.03 g
Potato & Garlic	3 slices	0.03 g
Mustangs	5 biscuits	2.58 g
Salticrax	3 biscuits	3.63 g
Savoy	5 biscuits	4.28 g
Wheatsworth	3 biscuits	3.30 g
RYVITA		
Dark	2 slices	0.30 g
Original	2 slices	0.28 g
Sesame	2 slices	1.26 g
VITAL		
Rice Cakes	2 slices	0.40 g

PRODUCT NAME	PORTION SIZE	FAT CONTENT (per serving)
WASA		
Crackerbread		
Crisp 'n Light Sourdough Rye	2 slices	0.00 g
Crisp 'n Light Wheat	2 slices	0.00 g
Crispbread		
Cinnamon Toast	2 slices	2.00 g
Fibre Rye	2 slices	2.00 g
Hearty Rye	2 slices	0.00 g
Light Rye	2 slices	0.00 g
Original Multi Grain	2 slices	0.00 g
Sourdough Rye	2 slices	0.00 g
Toasted Wheat with Sesame Seeds	2 slices	3.00 g
Wholewheat	2 slices	1.00 g
WEIGH-LESS		
Rice Cakes	2 slices	0.50 g
WOOLWORTHS		
Light Crisp Toasts	2 slices	2.00 g
Melba Toasts		
Cheese	2 slices	2.2 g
Herb & Pepper	2 slices	1.00 g
Multigrain	2 slices	1.00 g
Plain	2 slices	1.00 g
Rice Cakes		
Mini Apple & Cinnamon	5 cakes	0.40 g
Mini Blueberry Yoghurt	3 cakes	1.0 g
Mini Caramel Corn	5 cakes	0.20 g
Mini Carob	3 cakes	4.0 g
Mini Yoghurt	3 cakes	3.74 g
Oat & Sesame	2 slices	0.40 g
Plain	2 slices	0.20 g
Rice Crackers		
BBQ	5 crackers	1.29 g
Plain Salted	5 crackers	1.25 g
Sesame	5 crackers	1.05 g
Rye Crispbread	2 slices	0.20 g
Salted Crackers	3 biscuits	2.40 g
Salted Pretzels	⅓ packet	1.70 g
Savoury Biscuits		
Cheese	3 fingers	2.40 g
Sesame	3 fingers	4.20 g

PRODUCT NAME	PORTION SIZE	FAT CONTENT (per serving)
Sesame Crispbread	2 slices	2.40 g
Wholemeal Crispbread	2 slices	0.95 g

Other

PIRATE'S SNACKS

Salad Croûtons	1 tbsp	2.40 g

PANEALBA

Crostini Croûtons with Chilli	½ cup	3.50 g

DAIRY PRODUCTS

PRODUCT NAME	PORTION SIZE	FAT CONTENT (per serving)

Cheeses

CLOVER

Lichten Blanc Low Fat	matchbox size	4.5 g

FARMERS PRIDE

Cheese Powder	2 tbsp	3.2 g

HAPPY COW

Low-Fat Cheese Slices	1 slice	0.60 g

KRAFT

Philadelphia Fat-Free Cream Cheese	2 tbsp	0.00 g

MELROSE

Low-Fat Cheese Wedges	1 wedge	1.5 g

PICK 'N PAY CHOICE

Low-Fat Cottage Cheese	2 tbsp	1.5 g

RASKAS

Philadelphia Fat-Free Cream Cheese	2 tbsp	0.00 g

WOOLWORTHS

Fat-Free Cottage Cheese	2 tbsp	0.25 g
Low-Fat Cottage Cheese	2 tbsp	1.25 g
Reduced-Fat Cheddar (60%)	matchbox size	3.9 g

PRODUCT NAME	PORTION SIZE	FAT CONTENT (per serving)
Yoghurt & Milk Products		
DAIRYBELLE		
In Shape	1 small tub	0.50 g
Low-Fat Fruits of the Forest	1 small tub	3.50 g
Yoghurt Range	1 small tub	3.50 g
DAIRY GOLD		
Gero Diet		
Fat-Free	1 small tub	0.90 g
Low-Fat	1 small tub	3.50 g
DANONE		
Fruit Corners	1 tub	2.24 g
HOMESTEAD		
Low-Fat Fruit Yoghurt	1 small tub	2.63 g
PICK 'N PAY CHOICE		
Fat-Free Yoghurt Range	1 small tub	0.8 g
Low-Fat Yoghurt Range	1 small tub	2.5 g
Low-Fat Drinking Yoghurts	350 ml drink	5.0 g
Kiddies Layered Yoghurts	125 ml	2.57 g
ULTRA MEL		
Chocolate Milk	1 small carton	4.80 g
WOOLWORTHS		
Fat-Free Yoghurts	1 small tub	0.50 g
Fat-Free Drinking Yoghurts	250-ml bottle	0.80 g
Fat-Free Milk Shakes	300-ml bottle	1.50 g
Fat-Free Range Shape-Up	1 small tub	0.88 g
Go Kids Low-Fat Milks	200-ml bottle	3.40 g
Low-Fat Yoghurt Range		
Thick 'n Creamy	1 small tub	3.20 g
Thick 'n Fruity	1 small tub	2.60 g
Slimmer's Choice Range	1 small tub	0.90 g
Other Milk Products		
NESTLÉ		
Gold Medal Low-Fat Condensed Milk	2 tbsp	0.02 g
Ideal Milk Lite	¼ tin	3.50 g

PASTA, RICE AND POTATO DISHES

PRODUCT NAME	PORTION SIZE	FAT CONTENT (per serving)
Pasta & Sauces		
FATTI'S & MONI'S		
Suddenly Supper		
Beef Curry	⅙ packet	0.33 g
Bolognaise	⅙ packet	0.35 g
Farmstyle Casserole	⅙ packet	0.19 g
Ham Carbonara	⅙ packet	0.64 g
Mushroom & Garlic	⅙ packet	0.7 g
Tandoori Chicken	⅙ packet	0.52 g
NAPOLINA		
Alfredo	½ packet	3.2 g
Country Chicken & Mushroom	½ packet	3.3 g
Creamy Bacon Carbonara	½ packet	3.4 g
Roast Beef & Red Wine	½ packet	3.3 g
Wild Mushroom & Garlic	½ packet	3.3 g
PICK 'N PAY CHOICE		
Alfredo	½ packet	3.2 g
Macaroni Cheese	½ packet	4.7 g
Sour Cream & Chives	½ packet	3.1 g
Tomato & Herb	½ packet	2.5 g
ROYCO		
Alfredo	½ packet	1.52 g
Cheese, Ham & Mushroom	½ packet	1.91 g
Creamy Chicken, Parmesan & Herbs	½ packet	2.14 g
Creamy Bacon Carbonara	½ packet	1.16 g
Flavour Fiesta Range		
Hot Spicy Curry	½ packet	2.10 g
Mild Thai Curry	½ packet	1.80 g
Parmesan & Garlic	½ packet	2.20 g
Wild Mushroom, Garlic & Black Pepper	½ packet	1.60 g
Macaroni & Cheese	½ packet	2.20 g
Mince Mate		
3 Cheese	¼ packet	3.6 g
Boloroni	¼ packet	1.7 g
Creamy Cheese Noodles	¼ packet	3.0 g
Fruity Chutney Curry	¼ packet	1.5 g
Pizza Pasta	¼ packet	2.3 g

PRODUCT NAME	PORTION SIZE	FAT CONTENT (per serving)
Savaroni	¼ packet	1.8 g
Smokey Bacon 'n Chedda	¼ packet	3.0 g
Seafood Marinara	½ packet	1.00 g
Sour Cream & Chives	½ packet	0.75 g
Sour Cream & Mushroom	½ packet	0.50 g
Tuna Mate		
Chedda-melt	¼ packet	3.00 g
Lotsa Garlic & Herbs	¼ packet	2.10 g
More-ish Mushroom	¼ packet	1.60 g
Sunshine Tomato	¼ packet	2.30 g

Fresh Pasta
PICK 'N PAY CHOICE

3 Cheese Tortellini	½ packet	4.60 g
Beef Ravioli	½ packet	4.50 g
Beef Tortellini	½ packet	4.35 g
Chicken Ravioli	½ packet	4.00 g
Tagliatelle with Egg	½ packet	1.25 g

WOOLWORTHS

Tagliatelle	½ packet	1.75 g
Tagliolini	½ packet	1.44 g

Noodles
PICK 'N PAY

Choice Instant Noodles

Beef	1 packet	2.47 g
Chicken	1 packet	2.64 g
Curry	1 packet	3.33 g
Mushroom	1 packet	2.71 g
Shrimp	1 packet	3.18 g
Sweet & Sour Chicken	1 packet	3.54 g

Rice
TASTIC SAVOURY CLASSICS

Beef & Vegetable	¼ box	0.15 g
Beef Oriental	¼ box	0.21 g
Chicken a la Crème	¼ box	0.80 g
Peri-Peri Chicken	¼ box	0.40 g
Savoury Wild Rice	¼ box	0.08 g
Spicy Spanish	¼ box	0.40 g

PRODUCT NAME	PORTION SIZE	FAT CONTENT (per serving)
Summer Salad	¼ box	0.80 g
Wild Spinach & Onion	¼ box	1.35 g
Potato		
BROMOR FOODS		
Smash		
Country Herb	¼ packet	0.22 g
Garlic Butter	¼ packet	0.22 g
Original	¼ packet	0.22 g
Other		
BACHINI'S		
5-Minute Couscous	⅛ box	0.81 g

CONVENIENCE FOODS

PRODUCT NAME	PORTION SIZE	FAT CONTENT (per serving)
Frozen Foods		
CORAL LINE		
Potato Croquettes	3–4 croquettes	0.75 g
HEINZ		
Potato Slices/Chips	½ cup	4.70 g
Waffle Fries	½ cup	5.00 g
TODAY		
Pasta Shells in Italian-Style Tomato	½ tray	4.25 g
WEIGH-LESS		
Mediterranean Pizza	20-cm pizza	4.18 g
Oven Chips	½ cup	2.90 g
Paella	1 x 175-g tray	3.00 g
Spinach & Feta Pizza	20-cm pizza	4.36 g
WOOLWORTHS		
Frozen Mini Ham & Pineapple Pizzas	2 x 10-cm pizzas	3.90 g
Fresh Foods		
WOOLWORTHS		
Chargrilled Chicken Pasta	1 x 280-g tray	1.40 g

PRODUCT NAME	PORTION SIZE	FAT CONTENT (per serving)
Chicken & Vegetable Pie	1 x 350-g tray	3.15 g
Sweet 'n Sour Chicken with Egg-Fried Rice	1 x 350-g tray	2.45 g

FISH AND SEAFOOD

PRODUCT NAME	PORTION SIZE	FAT CONTENT (per serving)
Fresh Fish & Seafood		
WOOLWORTHS		
Smoked Mussels	¼ x 200-g tray	0.43 g
Frozen Fish & Seafood		
I & J		
Deepwater Hake Prime Steaks	1 steak	1.10 g
Fish Cakes	2 cakes	1.00 g
Haddock Fillets	1 fillet	1.38 g
Hake Portions – Extra Light	1 portion	4.10 g
Sliced Smoked Salmon	100 g	4.00 g
PICK 'N PAY CHOICE		
Calamari Rings	⅓ x 300-g box	trace
Choice Kingklip Steaks	1 steak	0.10 g
Haddock Mornay	¼ x 450-g box	3.82 g
New Zealand Mussels	⅓ x 300-g box	trace
Prawn Tails	⅓ x 300-g box	trace
Seafood Mix	⅓ x 300-g box	trace
Shrimps, cooked & peeled	⅓ x 300-g box	trace
Smoked Haddock in Rich Cheese	¼ x 450-g box	4.30 g
Sweet 'n Sour Hake	1 piece	1.65 g
SEA HARVEST		
Cape Whiting	1 fillet	1.10 g
Fish Cakes	2 cakes	2.30 g
Grill & Bakes		
Garlic & Herb	1 fillet	4.80 g
Lemon Pepper	1 fillet	4.85 g
Haddock Steaks	1 steak	1.40 g
Hake Fillets	1 fillet	3.00 g

PRODUCT NAME	PORTION SIZE	FAT CONTENT (per serving)
Hake Steaks	1 steak	1.20 g
Kingklip Fillets	1 fillet	0.12 g
WOOLWORTHS		
Calamari Rings	15 small rings	0.61 g
Char-Grilled Hake		
Garlic & Herb	1 portion	1.35 g
Lemon & Black Pepper	1 portion	1.35 g
Cocktail Prawns	10–12 prawns	0.20 g
Crab Sticks	7 sticks	0.23 g
Haddock Loins	1 loin	1.08 g
Haddock Steaks	1 steak	1.35 g
Hake Fillets/Loins	1 fillet	1.68 g
Hake Steaks	1 steak	2.10 g
Kabeljou Fillets	1 fillet	0.40 g
Kingklip Fillets/Steaks	1 fillet	0.90 g
Marinara Mix	½ cup	0.42 g
Yellowtail Fillets	1 fillet	0.40 g

Canned Fish & Seafood

PRODUCT NAME	PORTION SIZE	FAT CONTENT
ALL BRANDS		
Tuna in Brine	½ can	0.46 g
JOHN WEST		
Shrimps/Prawns in Brine	½ can	0.50 g
PICK 'N PAY CHOICE		
Tuna Chunks		
Curry Sauce with Vegetables & Pineapple	⅓ can	4.48 g
Mexican with Sweetcorn & Red Kidney Beans	⅓ can	0.22 g
Sweet & Sour with Vegetables & Pineapple	⅓ can	0.80 g

CHICKEN

PRODUCT NAME	PORTION SIZE	FAT CONTENT (per serving)
Fresh Chicken		
PICK 'N PAY CHOICE		
Cape Malay Sosaties	1 kebab	4.43 g
Indian Tikka Kebabs	1 kebab	1.89 g
Lemon & Black Pepper Kebabs	1 kebab	3.95 g
Peri-Peri Kebabs	1 kebab	1.94 g
WOOLWORTHS		
Char-Grilled Breast Fillets Peri-Peri	1 breast	3.20 g
Chicken Breast Mini Fillets		
Italian-Style Tomato Sauce	220 g	0.66 g
Sweet 'n Sour Pineapple Sauce	220 g	0.21 g
Chicken Roll	2 slices	3.80 g
Peri-Peri Chicken Bites	3 pieces	4.80 g
Shaved, Smoked Chicken	2 slices	0.60 g
Thai Kebabs	1 kebab	3.79 g
Tikka Chicken Breast Fillets	1 breast	1.77 g
Frozen Chicken		
TODAY		
Chicken Burgers	1 burger patty	4.20 g

MEAT

PRODUCT NAME	PORTION SIZE	FAT CONTENT (per serving)
Fresh Meat Products		
WOOLWORTHS		
Lean Bacon	3 rashers	1.30 g
Lean Smoked Ham	2 slices	0.80 g
Low-Fat Beef Burger Patties	1 burger patty	0.36 g
Shaved, Cooked Beef (wafer-thin)	2 slices	0.80 g
Shaved Turkey	2 slices	0.80 g

PRODUCT NAME	PORTION SIZE	FAT CONTENT (per serving)
Frozen Meat Products		
TODAY		
Burger Patties	1 burger patty	2.0 g

SALADS, FRUIT AND VEGETABLES

PRODUCT NAME	PORTION SIZE	FAT CONTENT (per serving)
Fresh Salads		
PICK 'N PAY FOODHALL		
Salad Packs		
Herb, Four Seasons	½ x 120-g pack	0.00 g
Medley	⅛ x 350-g pack	0.00 g
Sprout	¼ x 200-g pack	0.00 g
Salad Tubs		
French	½ x 300-g tub	0.00 g
Garden	½ x 300-g tub	0.00 g
WOOLWORTHS		
Salad Packs		
Californian	½ x 100-g pack	0.00 g
Sprout	½ x 100-g pack	0.00 g
Salad Tubs		
French.	½ x 210-g tub	0.00 g
Fresh Fruit		
KOO		
Froozee Fruit Festival	1 tub	0.00 g
Froozee Peach Paradise	1 tub	0.00 g
Froozee Pear Delights	1 tub	0.00 g
PICK 'N PAY CHOICE		
Fresh Fruit Salad	1 small tub	0.00 g
PICK 'N PAY FOODHALL		
Fresh Cut Fruit		
Fruit Salad	1 tub	0.00 g
Kiwifruit & Pineapple Pieces	1 tub	0.00 g
Melon Medley	1 tub	0.00 g
Pineapple Chunks	1 tub	0.00 g

PRODUCT NAME	PORTION SIZE	FAT CONTENT (per serving)
WOOLWORTHS		
Fresh Fruit Salad		
Seasonal	1 small tub	0.00 g
Winter Tropical	1 small tub	0.00 g
Frozen Fruit		
HILLCREST BERRY ORCHARDS		
Assorted Berries	¼ x 500-g bag	trace
PICK 'N PAY CHOICE		
Mixed Berries	¼ x 500-g tub	0.38 g
Dried Fruit		
SAFARI		
Assorted Fruit Flakes	½ x 100-g bag	0.15 g
Cling Peaches	2 halves	0.20 g
Dried Fruit Salad	3 halves	0.20 g
Frootz	¼ x 125-g bag	0.00 g
Sun-Dried Nectarines	2 halves	0.20 g
Sun-Dried Prunes	3 prunes	0.20 g
Sun-Dried Raisins & Sultanas	2 tbsp	0.10 g
WOOLWORTHS		
Dried Fruit Rolls	1 roll	0.00 g
Dried Peaches & Nectarines	¼ x 250-g bag	0.45 g
Dried Peeled Peaches	¼ x 250-g bag	0.45 g
Fruit Laces	1 x 25-g pack	0.00 g
Juicy Cubes		
Litchi/Pineapple/		
Mango/Granadilla	½ x 100-g bag	0.00 g
Mixed Dried Fruit	1 x 50-g pack	0.30 g
ZOAS PURE FOODS		
Pineapple Bites	⅓ bag	0.08 g
Papaya Bites/Mango Bites	⅓ bag	0.18 g
Fresh Vegetables		
PICK 'N PAY FOODHALL		
Asparagus with Butter	½ x 200-g pack	2.50 g
Baby Potatoes		
With Garlic Herb Butter	¼ x 400-g bag	2.50 g
With Spicy Butter	¼ x 400-g bag	2.50 g

PRODUCT NAME	PORTION SIZE	FAT CONTENT (per serving)
Fresh Soup Packs		
Butternut	¼ x 600 g	trace
Minestrone	¼ x 600 g	trace
Pea & Lentil	¼ x 600 g	trace
Vegetable	¼ x 600 g	trace
Mediterranean Vegetable Kebabs	1 kebab	3.00 g
Mix of Four Vegetables	1 cup	0.00 g
Stir-Fries		
Country	½ x 600-g tray	0.00 g
Plain	½ x 600-g tray	0.00 g
With Pasta	½ x 600-g tray	trace
Stuffed Butternut		
Spinach & Feta	½ large butternut	3.75 g
WOOLWORTHS		
Char-Grilled Roast Vegetables	½ tray	3.00 g
Filled Butternut		
Spinach, Mushroom, Feta	½ large butternut	2.80 g
Sweet Potato & Cinnamon	½ large butternut	4.20 g
Stir-Fries		
Chinese Sweet 'n Spicy	1 x 230 g-tray	0.70 g
Chow Mein	½ x 500-g tray	3.64 g
Oriental	½ x 500-g tray	trace
Ribbon Vegetable	½ x 500-g tray	trace
Seasonal	½ x 500-g tray	trace
Vegetable & Pineapple	½ x 500-g tray	trace
With Sweet 'n Sour Sauce	⅓ x 500-g tray	0.30 g
Veg 'n Sauce		
Butternut, Courgette, Spinach with Tomato & Onion Sauce	½ tray	0.70 g
Mixed Vegetables & Creamy Curry	½ tray	3.30 g
Frozen Vegetables		
PICK 'N PAY CHOICE		
Stir-Fries		
Chinese	1–2 cups	2.00 g
Italian; Garden Mix	1–2 cups	trace
Mushroom	1–2 cups	1.00 g
TABLE TOP		
Stir-Fries		
Garden Mix	1–2 cups	1.00 g

PRODUCT NAME	PORTION SIZE	FAT CONTENT (per serving)
Hawaiian Mix	1–2 cups	0.70 g
Oriental Mix	1–2 cups	1.00 g

SOUPS, SAUCES, DRESSINGS, MARINADES AND GRAVIES

PRODUCT NAME	PORTION SIZE	FAT CONTENT (per serving)
Fresh Soups		
DENNY		
Soup of the Day		
Cream of Mushroom	1 cup	1.80 g
Mushroom & Chicken	1 cup	2.30 g
Mushroom & Vegetable	1 cup	0.3 g
Mushroom, Leek & Asparagus	1 cup	2.50 g
PICK 'N PAY FOODHALL		
Butternut	1 cup = ½ pack	4.85 g
SMITH & HOSKIN		
Dining-In Soups		
Chinese Chicken & Corn	½ pack	2.48 g
Tuscan Bean & Pasta	½ pack	0.68 g
WOOLWORTHS		
Carrot & Coriander	1 cup	1.00 g
Italian Bean & Tomato	1 cup	0.70 g
Instant Soups		
BAXTERS		
Healthy Choice Canned Soups		
Autumn Vegetable	½ can	0.40 g
Carrot, Onion & Chickpea	½ can	0.20 g
Chicken & Sweetcorn	½ can	2.6 g
Chicken & Vegetable	½ can	1.10 g
Chicken & Wild Korma Spice	½ can	4.30 g
Country Garden	½ can	1.10 g
French Onion	½ can	0.20 g
Italian Tomato with Basil	½ can	3.00 g
Mushroom	½ can	3.40 g

PRODUCT NAME	PORTION SIZE	FAT CONTENT (per serving)
Potato & Leek	½ can	0.40 g
Spicy Tomato & Rice		
with Sweetcorn	½ can	0.60 g
HEINZ		
Canned Soup		
Wholesome Lentil	½ can	0.40 g
MAGGI		
Soup Drinks	¼ packet	3.92 g
PICK 'N PAY		
Choice		
Country Vegetable	½ can	0.25 g
Superb Instant Soups with Croûtons	⅓ packet	2.85 g
ROYCO		
Cup-a-Soup		
Chicken Noodle	1 sachet	1.80 g
Hearty Beef	1 sachet	0.90 g
Mushroom	1 sachet	1.60 g
Cup-a-Soup Lite	1 sachet	0.90 g
Mexican Tomato	1 sachet	2.60 g
Supreme with Croûtons	1 sachet	2.30 g

Sauces

ALL GOLD READY-TO-EAT		
Cook-In-Sauces		
Creamy White Wine	¼ can	trace
Red Wine & Herbs	¼ can	trace
Spicy Curry	¼ can	trace
Sweet 'n Sour	¼ can	trace
Potato Bake		
Cheese & French Onion	¼ pack	1.00 g
Smokey Bacon & Golden Cheese	¼ pack	0.90 g
AMOY		
Black Bean Stir-Fry Sauce	½ sachet	0.15 g
Black Pepper Sauce	½ sachet	2.85 g
Lemon Sauce	½ sachet	0.08 g
Plum Stir-Fry Sauce	½ sachet	0.08 g
Sweet 'n Sour Sauce	½ sachet	0.15 g
Yellow Bean Stir-Fry Sauce	½ sachet	0.25 g
DENNY SAUCES		
Garlic Mushroom	⅓ can	1.9 g

PRODUCT NAME	PORTION SIZE	FAT CONTENT (per serving)
Pepper Mushroom	⅓ can	2.4 g
HASTY TASTY SAUCES		
Sweet 'n Sour	N/A	0.00 g
Sweet 'n Sour Braai	N/A	0.00 g
INA PAARMAN		
Apple & Soy Sauce	¼ cup	< 5 g
Spicy Curry Sauce	¼ cup	5.00 g
PICK 'N PAY FOODHALL		
Fresh Sauces		
Cheese	¼ pack	5.00 g
Mushroom	¼ pack	3.10 g
Pepper	¼ pack	4.20 g
ROYCO PACKET SAUCES		
Cheddar Cheese	¼ cup	0.97 g
Creamy Mushroom	¼ cup	1.31 g
Potato Bake	¼ packet	1.00 g
Sweet 'n Sour	¼ cup	0.13 g
White	¼ cup	0.61 g
SMITH & HOSKIN		
Dining In		
Chinese Sweet 'n Sour	¼ pack	2.36 g
STEERS		
BBQ; Peri-Peri	2 tbsp	trace
WALNUT RIDGE		
Incredible Casserole		
Brewers Beef Stew	¼ pack	3.88 g
Creamy Stroganoff	¼ pack	4.38 g
Farmers Country Casserole	¼ pack	2.75 g
Tomato Bredie	¼ pack	0.63 g
Irresistible Curry		
Mild Fruity Curry	½ cup	3.63 g
Mmm ... Fresh Sauces		
Chunky Mushroom	¼ cup	2.19 g
Creamy Cheese	¼ cup	1.40 g
Ground Peppercorn	¼ cup	4.25 g
Unbelievable Chicken		
Hawaiian Pineapple	¼ pack	0.38 g
Savoury Farmstyle Apricot	¼ pack	0.38 g
WEIGH-LESS		
Mushroom	¼ cup	0.45 g

PRODUCT NAME	PORTION SIZE	FAT CONTENT (per serving)
Pepper	¼ cup	0.45 g
WOOLWORTHS		
Cook-In-Sauces		
Cape Malay Curry	¼ can	4.5 g
Durban Curry	¼ can	2.05 g
Mediterranean Tomato	¼ can	2.56 g
Mushroom & White Wine	¼ can	4.10 g
Oriental Sweet 'n Sour	¼ can	0.10 g
Red Wine & Herb	¼ can	0.30 g
Fresh Orange & Cranberry Sauce	¼ pack	0.68 g
Fresh Sweet 'n Sour Sauce	½ pack	0.10 g
Grill & Bake Sauces		
Sweet & Spicy	¼ pack	4.70 g
Sauces for Vegetables		
Pineapple & Lemon	½ pack	0.30 g
Sweet 'n Sour	½ pack	0.30 g
Pasta Sauces		
PICK 'N PAY CHOICE		
Italian Classic		
Arrabiatta	¼ bottle	4.20 g
Garlic	¼ bottle	3.08 g
Original	¼ bottle	3.08 g
Passata	⅛ bottle	trace
Pepper	¼ bottle	2.94 g
Premium Pasta Sauces		
Basil & Olive Oil	½ bottle	4.05 g
Garlic & Oreganum	½ bottle	4.05 g
ROYCO		
Bacon Carbonara	⅓ cup	3.00 g
Cheese, Ham & Mushroom	⅓ cup	2.70 g
Creamy Cheese & Garlic	⅓ cup	3.30 g
Creamy Herb & Tomato	⅓ cup	3.00 g
Sour Cream & Mushroom	⅓ cup	2.10 g
Tomato & Bacon	⅓ cup	2.20 g
WALNUT RIDGE		
Garden Red Pepper	¼ pack	0.6 g
Mediterranean Olive & Tomato	¼ pack	1.9 g
Tomato & Basil	¼ pack	0.1 g

PRODUCT NAME	PORTION SIZE	FAT CONTENT (per serving)
WOOLWORTHS		
Bottled Pasta Sauces		
Hot Salsa	½ cup	1.25 g
Italian Tomato Purée	⅙ bottle	0.60 g
Tomato & Herb	½ cup	0.40 g
Tomato, Garlic & Basil	¼ bottle	4.50 g
Fresh Pasta Sauces		
Char-Grilled Veg in Tomato Sauce	½ pack	4.00 g

Salad Dressings

PRODUCT NAME	PORTION SIZE	FAT CONTENT (per serving)
ALL JOY		
Figure No-Oil Dressings	2 tsp	0.00 g
CROSSE & BLACKWELL		
Trim Mayonnaise	1 tbsp	1.60 g
Waistline Fat-Free Dressings		
Greek, French,	1 tbsp	0.00 g
Italian, Mexican	1 tbsp	1.60 g
HEINZ FAT-FREE DRESSINGS		
Buttermilk Ranch	1 sachet	0.00 g
Honey Dijon	1 sachet	0.00 g
Parmesan & Peppercorn	1 sachet	0.00 g
Thousand Islands	1 sachet	0.00 g
HELLMANS		
Light Mayonnaise	1 tbsp	4.52 g
INA PAARMAN		
Low-Oil Dressings		
French	1 tbsp	1.10 g
Italian, Greek	1 tbsp	0.70 g
KNORR		
Light Oil-Free Range	1 tbsp	0.00 g
ROYCO		
Fat-Free Dressings		
Greek, French, Italian	1 tbsp	0.00 g
Lite Creamy Dressings		
Blue Cheese, Four Seasons	1 tbsp	1.70 g
Thousand Islands	1 tbsp	1.70 g
WEIGH-LESS		
Low-Oil Dressings	1 tbsp	2.00 g
WOOLWORTHS		
Lemon & Basil Dressing	2 tbsp	1.25 g

PRODUCT NAME	PORTION SIZE	FAT CONTENT (per serving)
Low-Oil Dressings		
Greek, Italian, French	2 tbsp	2.9 g
Roasted Pepper Dressing	2 tbsp	1.00 g

Marinades
ALL JOY
Before You Braai Basting Sauces & Marinades		
Chicken	2 tbsp	1.50 g
Meat	2 tbsp	1.50 g

HEINZ
BBQ Cajun-Style	2 tbsp	0.00 g
BBQ Honey & Mustard	2 tbsp	0.00 g
Buffalo Wing	2 tbsp	0.00 g

INA PAARMAN
Marinate-in-a-Bag		
Green Peppercorn	¼ packet	2.28 g
Honey & Soy	¼ packet	1.70 g
Italian Tomato	¼ packet	2.60 g
Rosemary & Mint	1¼ packet	2.23 g

KNORR
Spare Rib	¼ packet	trace
Tropical Fruit	¼ packet	trace

ROBERTSONS BAGS-OF-FLAVOUR
Blackened Cajun	½ sachet	0.35 g
Honey BBQ	½ sachet	0.20 g
Mushroom & Onion	½ sachet	0.30 g
Spicy BBQ	½ sachet	0.15 g
Sweet 'n Sour	½ sachet	0.05 g

ROYCO
Chicken Marinade	¼ packet	< 5 g
Garlic Steak Marinade	¼ packet	< 5 g

STEERS
Chicken	N/A	trace
Steakmaker	N/A	trace

WOOLWORTHS
Chicken	N/A	trace
Meat	N/A	trace

PRODUCT NAME	PORTION SIZE	FAT CONTENT (per serving)
Gravies		
COLMAN'S		
Oxo Chicken Gravy	¼ packet	0.58 g
Oxo Lamb Gravy	¼ packet	0.46 g
PICK 'N PAY FOODHALL		
Rich Brown Gravy	¼ packet	2.5 g
ROYCO		
Brown Onion	¼ packet	0.55 g
Rich Savoury	¼ packet	0.70 g
Roast Chicken	¼ packet	0.65 g
Roast Meat	¼ packet	0.86 g
WALNUT RIDGE		
Roast Chicken Gravy	¼ packet	0.30 g
Roast Meat Gravy	¼ packet	1.80 g
WEIGH-LESS		
Chicken Gravy	¼ packet	0.85 g
Rich Beef Gravy	¼ packet	0.45 g
WOOLWORTHS		
Rich Brown Gravy	¼ packet	1.25 g
Roast Poultry Gravy	¼ packet	1.90 g

MISCELLANEOUS

PRODUCT NAME	PORTION SIZE	FAT CONTENT (per serving)
Condiments		
CARMEL		
Good 'n Chunky Sauces		
Tomato; Mustard; BBQ	N/A	trace
CROSSE & BLACKWELL		
Chilli & Garlic Sauce	1 tbsp	0.05 g
Chilli Sauce	1 tbsp	trace
Salsa Sauce	1 tbsp	trace
HP FOODS		
HP Sauce	1 tbsp	trace

PRODUCT NAME	PORTION SIZE	FAT CONTENT (per serving)
WELLINGTON		
Chilli Sauces		
Sweet; Hot; Garlic	1 tbsp	trace
Chunky Chutney		
Mild; Hot; Extra Hot; Mint;		
Sultana; Ginger	1 tbsp	0.00 g

Coatings & Flavourings

PRODUCT NAME	PORTION SIZE	FAT CONTENT (per serving)
ALL GOLD		
Fresh Cut, Diced, Peeled Tomato		
Garlic, Basil & Origanum	¼–½ can	trace
Natural	¼–½ can	trace
Onion & Garlic	¼–½ can	trace
BOKOMO		
Spicy Chicken Breadcrumbs	N/A	0.00 g
BUTTER BUDS		
Sprinkles – Butter Flavouring	1 tbsp	0.00 g
GOLDCREST		
Coconut Milk	¼ cup	3.00 g
BAC-OS		
Bacon-Flavoured Chips	1 tbsp	1.50 g
HINDS SOUTHERN FRIED COATING		
Chilli; Hot	N/A	< 5 g
Lemon Herb	N/A	< 5 g
KELLOGGS CORNFLAKE CRUMBS		
BBQ; Regular; Seasoned; Peri-Peri	N/A	0.00 g
MRS MANISCHEWITZ		
Potato Roasters – Herb & Garlic	1 tbsp	0.50 g
PICK 'N PAY CHOICE ITALIAN CLASSIC		
Chopped Peeled Tomatoes		
For Bolognaise	¼–½ can	trace
With Basil	¼–½ can	0.35 g
With Chilli	¼–½ can	trace
With Garlic	¼–½ can	trace
With Herbs	¼–½ can	0.23 g
With Peppers & Onion	¼–½ can	1.05 g
ROKEACH		
Shakin' Potatoes		
Country; BBQ	1 tbsp	0.50 g

PRODUCT NAME	PORTION SIZE	FAT CONTENT (per serving)
SPAR		
Chopped Italian Tomato & Mushroom	¼–½ can	0.10 g
Chopped Italian Tomato & Onion	¼–½ can	0.20 g

Pizza Toppings
PICK 'N PAY CHOICE

Italian Classic Pizza Topping		
With Herbs	¼ bottle	0.63 g
With Mushrooms	¼ bottle	0.68 g
With Olives	¼ bottle	0.63 g
With Peppers	¼ bottle	0.53 g

Spreads
CROSSE & BLACKWELL

Sandwich Spread	2 tsp	2.46 g
HEINZ		
Sandwich Spread	2 tsp	1.3 g
MELROSE		
Low-Fat Cheese Spread	1 tbsp	1.5 g
NAPOLINA		
Over The Top	2 tsp	0.3 g
NESTLÉ		
Lite Cheese Spread	2 tsp	1.0 g
PECK'S		
Anchovette	1 tsp	trace
Beef 'n Biltong	1 tsp	trace
Chicken Liver	1 tsp	trace
Chicken Tikka	1 tsp	trace
Vegetarian	1 tsp	trace
REDRO		
Anchovy Paste	1 tsp	0.00 g
ROBERTSONS		
Beefy Bovril/Marmite	1 tsp	0.00 g
UNIFOODS		
Oxo	1 tsp	0.00 g

Jams
All jams & fruit spreads, honey and syrup	1 tsp	0.00 g

PRODUCT NAME	PORTION SIZE	FAT CONTENT (per serving)
Dips and Starters		
BAKER STREET		
Snack Dips		
Cheese & Chives	2 tbsp	0.30 g
Garlic & Cucumber	(prepared	0.30 g
Peppercorn	with fat-free	0.30 g
Spring Onion	cottage cheese)	0.30 g
CUBBS PARTY DIPS		
Bacon & Onion	2 tbsp	0.00 g
Garlic & Tangy Tomato	(prepared	4.00 g
Onion & Garlic	with	0.00 g
Smoked Ham & Cheese	fat-free	5.00 g
Sour Cream & Spring Onion	cottage cheese)	4.00 g
KRAFT		
Assorted Dips	2 tbsp	< 5 g
PICK 'N PAY FOODHALL		
Greek Keftedes	2–3	4.20 g
Mexican Dip Selection – Salsa	2 tbsp	0.90 g
Tzatziki	2 tbsp	2.00 g
Mexican Range		
OLD EL PASO		
Burrito Tortilla	1 large tortilla	4.8 g
Cheese & Salsa	2 tbsp	3.00 g
Enchilada Tortilla	1 small tortilla	2.6 g
Enchilada Sauce	2 heaped tbsp	0.10 g
Refried Beans	¾ cup	0.5 g
Salsa	4 heaped tbsp	0.00 g
Taco Sauce	2 heaped tbsp	0.00 g
Other		
COLMAN FOODS		
Spray and Cook	N/A	0.00 g
OLIVE GROVE		
Olive oil spray	5 g = 1 application	3.50 g
SPANJAARD LTD		
Antonio's Cook 'n Bake		
Olive Oil	5 g = 1 application	2.50 g
Original	5 g = 1 application	2.50 g

SWEET TREATS

PRODUCT NAME	PORTION SIZE	FAT CONTENT (per serving)
Chilled Desserts		
ALL BRANDS		
Jelly	¼ packet	0.00 g
DELITE FOODS		
Instant Chocolate Mousse	¼ packet	1.90 g
FARMERS PRIDE		
Instant Milk Tart Mix		
(using skim milk)	1 wedge	0.76 g
MOIR'S		
Crème Caramel	¼ packet	trace
PICK 'N PAY FOODHALL		
Flavoured Custards	½ x 250-ml tub	3.65 g
Jelly & Custard – three flavours	1 x 120-g tub	0.62 g
Crème Caramel	1 x 125 ml	< 5 g
ROYAL		
Crème Caramel	⅙ packet	trace
WOOLWORTHS		
Fruit Jelly	1 x 180-g tub	0.00 g
Go Kidz Range		
Jelly with Cosmic Bits	1 x 150-g tub	1.50 g
Layered Custard Dessert	1 x 125-ml tub	2.68 g
Jelly & Custard	1 x 90-g tub	0.50 g
Frozen Desserts		
CAS ICE CREAM		
Diaby	100 ml	2.90 g
DAIRY DELITE		
Fruit Pops	1 lolly	0.00 g
DUN ROBIN		
Dairy Soft	100 ml	1.80 g
Guilt-free	100 ml	< 1 g
LIQUIFRUIT	1 lolly	0.00 g
NESTLÉ		
Dairymaid Country Fresh Lite	100 ml	2.30 g
OLA		
Diet Delight	100 ml	3.10 g
WEIGH-LESS		
Vanilla Dairy Dessert	½ cup	3.94 g

PRODUCT NAME	PORTION SIZE	FAT CONTENT (per serving)
WOOLWORTHS		
Frozen Fruit Shells	1 shell	0.00 g
Frozen Yoghurt	1 medium scoop	3.76 g
Slimmers Choice Frozen Dessert	1 medium scoop	2.00 g

Dessert Toppings & Sauces

PRODUCT NAME	PORTION SIZE	FAT CONTENT
ALL JOY		
Kiddies Chocolate Sauce	1 tbsp	0.00 g
BONNITA		
Ready-to-Eat Custard	½ cup	3.38 g
BORDEN FOODS		
Instant Custard	½ cup	< 5 g
CHEF'S CHOICE		
Chocodero Sauces	1 tbsp	< 5 g
CLOVER		
Ultramel Custard	½ cup	3.90 g
Ultramel Lite Custard	½ cup	2.13 g
CRUSHA		
Sauce / Milkshake Mix		
Chocolate	2–3 tbsp	0.76 g
Vanilla, Strawberry, Fruit	1–2 tbsp	0.00 g
ILLOVO		
Finest Chocolate Sauce	2 tbsp	0.30 g
INA PAARMAN		
Caramel, Mint, Strawberry,		
Orange, Coffee	2 tbsp	2.60 g
MOIR'S		
Instant Custard	½ cup	< 5 g
Quick & Easy Creamo	100 ml prepared	1.32 g
ORLEY FOODS		
Orley Whip Lite	¼ sachet	4.18 g
ROBERTSONS		
Original Chocolate Sauce	1 tbsp	0.00 g
Really Really Rich Sauces	1 tbsp	0.00 g
TATE & LYLE		
Tops Flavoured Syrups	1 tbsp	0.00 g
WOOLWORTHS		
Berry Dessert Sauce	2 tbsp	0.18 g
Fat-Reduced Cream	2 tbsp	4.50 g
Fruit Toppings	4 tbsp	0.00 g

PRODUCT NAME	PORTION SIZE	FAT CONTENT (per serving)
Vanilla Custard (UHT)	100 ml	4.00 g

Sweets

BEACON
Bananas	3 x each	0.00 g
Boiled Sweets		
Fruit Salad	3 x each	0.30 g
Sparkles	3 x each	0.00 g
Dr Bean Jelly Beans	6 x each	0.00 g
Dr Bean Jelly Juices	6 x each	0.00 g
Liquorice Allsorts	3 x each	0.90 g
Manhattan's Marshmallows	6 x each	0.00 g
Sour Worms	3 worms	0.00 g

MR SWEET
Snakes Alive	3 x each	0.00 g

WEIGH-LESS
Fruit Gums	1 x 40-g packet	trace

WILSONS
Mint Imperials	3 x each	0.00 g

SNACKS

PRODUCT NAME	PORTION SIZE	FAT CONTENT (per serving)

Milk Drinks

ALL JOY
Hot Chok	2 tbsp	1.80 g

CLIFTON
Hot Chok	2 tbsp	1.80 g
Mint Chok	2 tbsp	1.80 g

NESTLÉ
Bar One	2 tbsp	0.60 g
Hot Chocolate	2 tbsp	2.20 g
Milo	2 tbsp	2.00 g
Nesquick	1 tbsp	0.42 g

SMITHKLINE BEECHAM
Horlicks Chocolate	2 tbsp	0.70 g

PRODUCT NAME	PORTION SIZE	FAT CONTENT (per serving)
SWISS MISS		
Lite Hot Cocoa Mix	1 sachet	1.00 g
WANDER FOODS		
Ovaltine	2 tbsp	1.20 g
WOOLWORTHS		
Hot Chocolate	2 tbsp	1.80 g

Savoury Snacks

BAKER STREET		
Pretzola Mini Pretzels		
Flavoured	1 small packet	5.00 g
Lightly Salted, Marmite	1 small packet	5.00 g
GOLDEN VALLEY		
Act 2 Micro Popcorn	½ packet	4.50 g
LA BICI		
Pasta Snacks		
Pepper Salami	¼ box	4.50 g
Spicy BBQ	¼ box	4.50 g
Vinegar & Lemon	¼ box	4.50 g
PIRATE'S		
Rice Crisps		
Golden Sesame	¼ box	2.51 g
Lightly Salted	¼ box	3.11 g
Pink shrimp	¼ box	3.30 g
SNAXELS		
Pretzels	⅓ bag	< 5 g
WEIGH-LESS		
Cheddar Snacks	1 small packet	4.70 g
Beef Biltong Sticks	1 small packet	5.00 g
WILLARDS		
Flings	1 small packet	3.0 g
WOOLWORTHS		
Beef Biltong – sliced	¼ pack	1.92 g
Crisp Beef Biltong Chips	¼ pack	2.40 g
Crisp Beef Biltong Snapsticks	¼ pack	1.70 g

PRODUCT NAME	PORTION SIZE	FAT CONTENT (per serving)
Snack Bars		
BARRY'S		
Peanut Power; Fruit 7 Nut	55-g bar	(no
Yog Nut; Yoghurt Fruit Muesli	65-g bar	added
Yoghurt Muesli	60-g bar	fat)
Chocolate Fruit & Nut	60-g bar	0.00 g
Granola	55-g bar	0.00 g
Slim Snack	55-g bar	(no added
Nougat Nut; Nougat Fruit & Nut	70-g bar	fat)
GILLY		
Peach & Pineapple Yoghurt Bar	45-g bar	3.00 g
Raisin & Grape Yoghurt Bar	45-g bar	3.00 g
KELLOGGS		
Nutrigrain	37-g bar	3.00 g
Rice Crispy Treats	37-g bar	3.50 g
SAD		
Just Fruit	32-g bar	0.10 g
WEIGH-LESS		
Apple Wheat Bar	20-g bar	3.12 g
Fruit & Yoghurt Cereal Bar	20-g bar	3.32 g
WOOLWORTHS		
Orange & Lemon Bar	50-g bar	4.90 g

CHAPTER THREE

Preparing Low-Fat Meals At Home

COMMONLY ASKED QUESTIONS AND USEFUL COOKING TIPS

The following are questions that I am often asked by clients in my dietetic practice. They are all valid queries, as even I was taught that if I want to make a white sauce, for example, I first need to make a roux using margarine and milk. Here you will find useful tips for making a white sauce without margarine, stir-frying without using oil, and much more.

MAIN DISHES

How can I make microwaved vegetables tasty without adding butter?
- ❖ Place the washed vegetables in a microwave dish with a dash of water, sprinkle over vegetable stock and microwave until *al dente*.
- ❖ Cook the vegetables as described above, omitting the stock. When the vegetables are cooked, drizzle with lemon juice and serve.

How do I make a stir-fry without using oil?
- ❖ When you are browning the meat, chicken or vegetables, use beef, chicken or vegetable stock and add water, wine, sherry, fruit or vegetable juices when you need to add liquid.
- ❖ Even an egg can be fried using just Spray and Cook.
- ❖ A non-stick frying pan is very useful.

I know cheese is high in fat – how can I achieve a nice cheesy flavour using less fat?
- ❖ Use Parmesan, extra mature Cheddar cheese or cheese powder – you will need much less cheese to get the same cheesy flavour.
- ❖ Try using low-fat cheese spread or wedges on pizzas or sandwiches.

What can I use instead of pastry when making pies and quiches?
- ❖ Phyllo pastry is a convenient, easy-to-use, low-fat option.
- ❖ Try mixing mashed potato/cooked rice and egg-white – one cup of potato or rice to one-egg white – to create a base. Bake the base for 10 minutes in a moderate oven before adding the filling.

What can I use instead of salad dressings?
- ❖ Balsamic vinegar
- ❖ Lemon juice and herbs
- ❖ Make a dressing combining tomato or vegetable juice, vinegar, herbs and sugar.
- ❖ Make a mayonnaise using fat-free plain yoghurt, mustard and honey, or add your own flavourings.

How can I make a 'legal' pizza?
- ❖ Make your own or buy ready-made pizza bases and spread with a tomato and onion purée mix and fresh herbs.
- ❖ The following ingredients can all be used: ham, pineapple, banana, chopped chicken breast, seafood, anchovies, garlic, mushrooms, asparagus, spinach and peppers or chilli.
- ❖ Add no mozzarella or other yellow cheeses – a sprinkling of either feta, Parmesan or extra-mature Cheddar cheese can be added on top, as very little of these cheeses is needed to achieve a strong cheese flavour.

How can I make a fat-free white sauce?
- ❖ Heat 1 cup fat-free milk, removing it from the heat just before it comes to the boil. Separately, mix about 2–3 tsp cornflour in half a cup of cold milk to form a paste. Stirring constantly, add some of the cold paste to the hot milk, and bring the mixture to the boil. Keep adding more paste until you achieve the desired consistency. Add flavouring such as herbs, mustard powder, stock powder, spices, or cheese.

How can I brown onions without using fat?
- ❖ Toss the chopped onions into a pan without any liquid and allow to cook until they are just starting to stick and go brown. Now add a little water, sherry, stock or wine, and hey presto – brown onions!

What can I use instead of cream to make cream sauces?

❖ Low-fat evaporated milk

❖ Buttermilk

❖ Fat-free plain yoghurt

Make sure that the buttermilk or yoghurt is added just before serving, as bringing either of these ingredients to the boil will result in the sauce curdling.

What do I use as a baste for roast meat to stop it from drying out?

❖ Put the joint on a grill over a dish half-filled with water – this allows the fat from the meat to drip into the dish and the steam from the dish prevents the joint from drying out.

❖ If you are roasting a chicken breast or a piece of fish, baste it using a dressing such as lemon juice and sherry or wine, or soy sauce and honey, and then wrap it in tinfoil to prevent it from drying out.

❖ Chicken or even fish can be roasted in the Spanish tradition by placing the whole chicken in a casserole dish, and coating it completely it in a layer of coarse salt – use 2 bags (2 kg) of coarse salt per chicken. After baking in the oven for approximately 1½ hours, the salt will have formed a fatty crust that can be broken away to leave a very tasty low-fat meal.

I usually fry my pork chops. How else can I cook them?

❖ For 2 small chops, make a basting sauce using 1 tsp Trim mayonnaise and 1 tsp chutney. Grill the chops, allowing the excess fat to drip into a dripping tray.

❖ Remember to remove all excess fat from the chops before cooking.

SNACKS

What can I use instead of butter or margarine?

❖ Low-fat or fat-free smooth cottage cheese can be used as a delicious spread on bread or bread substitutes.

❖ Flora Extra Light spread is recommended.

❖ Use mustard for meat sandwiches, and pickles or chutney for cheese sandwiches.

❖ Low-fat salad cream is great for chicken, tuna or egg sandwiches.

What can be used as low-fat sandwich fillings or toast toppings?

❖ Mashed banana – try topping it with Marmite or chutney
❖ Fat-free or low-fat cottage cheese – either smooth or chunky – and add pickles or fresh herbs, sunflower seeds, or fresh fruit like banana, pineapple, etc.
❖ Lean ham or beef with mustard and pickles
❖ Smoked, shaved ham, chicken or turkey with salad and a thin scraping of low-fat mayonnaise or mustard
❖ Fat-free cream cheese – as a decadent treat
❖ Fishpaste or sandwich spread
❖ Bovril or Marmite
❖ Jam, marmalade or honey – try cottage cheese, honey and sunflower seeds
❖ Low-fat cheese wedges or low-fat cheese spread

Can you suggest some good snacks?

❖ Fresh or dried fruit
❖ Salads with fat-free dressings – try Sue Long's strawberry dressing
❖ Soups – especially home-made or convenient lite instant soups
❖ Fat-free yoghurts
❖ Boudoir biscuits
❖ Low-fat crackers or bread sticks dipped in cottage cheese
❖ Vegetable sticks
❖ Dry popped popcorn flavoured with lemon juice and salt, or even Aromat or chicken spice

Which snack bars are low in fat?

❖ Barry's Fruit and Nut, Slim Snack or Nougat Fruit & Nut bar
❖ Kelloggs Rice Krispy Treats or Nutrigrain bars
❖ Weigh-less Apple Wheat or Fruit & Yoghurt Cereal bar
❖ SAD Just Fruit bars

DESSERTS OR BAKING

What can I use instead of cream cheese in desserts like Pavlova and cheesecake?

❖ Use fat-free smooth cottage cheese – it can be thinned down with buttermilk or fat-free plain yoghurt.

How can I reduce the fat content of my favourite muffin, bread or cake recipe?
❖ Use fruit purée or buttermilk to replace half the oil or margarine.

How can I garnish desserts that are traditionally garnished with cream or ice cream?
❖ Use low-fat or fat-free ice cream or a sorbet or low-fat frozen yoghurt.
❖ Use fresh herbs (like mint), fruit slices or edible flowers (like pansies and nasturtiums).

How can I make fat-free custard?
❖ Follow the instructions on the instant custard powder container, but use fat-free milk instead of full-cream milk.
❖ Artificial sweeteners can be used instead of sugar.

SUITABLE RECIPES

The following recipes have been collected from various sources and tested by family, friends and clients from Karen Protheroe's Dietetic Practices at six different Health & Racquet Clubs.

There is a range in the number of servings produced from each recipe. This is to accommodate the appetite, age, gender and activity levels of those eating the recipe meal. It is clear that a recipe which serves 4–6 would provide enough food for either 4 hungry athletes or 6 small eaters.

Nutritional analysis of recipes per portion was done using a Dietetic Software Programme designed by the Medical Research Council. Due to the constant emergence of new foodstuffs, it was, at times, necessary to make comparative estimates in order to calculate the nutritional contri-bution of the recipe. When calculating the nutritional information per portion, an average of the recipe yield was used. For example, the Hummus recipe (*see* page 83) serves 4–6, so an average of 5 was used for the analysis. This information is thus a guide to the nutritional contri-bution per portion of each recipe.

For those readers with time or other constraints, most of the recipes given here are followed by a list of one or more quick convenience foods that may be used as alternatives. The convenience foods are included in the shopping lists given in Chapter Two (*see* pages 31–65), and this also means that the relevant nutritional information is immediately available.

Each recipe has also been evaluated in terms of its suitability for individuals with particular requirements. The recipes may fulfil one or more of the following requirements: be suitable for vegetarians, for those with heart concerns, for diabetics, and for microwave cooking. Brief explanations of the categories are given below:

VEGETARIAN

These recipes are suitable for lacto-ovo vegetarians who eat egg and dairy products. Some recipes may also contain other animal products, including gelatine, Worcestershire sauce or fish sauce. Strict vegans would thus not necessarily be able to use all the recipes in this category.

HEART SMART

It must be noted that although recipes have been analysed and selected on the grounds of being low in fat, the fat source has not been considered. For example, no distinction has been made between whether the fat is saturated, monounsaturated or otherwise.

DIABETIC

These recipes are suitable for diabetics with controlled blood sugar levels, who may as part of a meal consume small amounts of sucrose (table sugar). By being low in fat, their suitability for diabetics is further enhanced.

MICROWAVE

Recipes in this category are suitable for preparation in a microwave oven. Cooking times may need to be adjusted in order to accommodate the variability in the wattage or power output of different ovens.

If you are unsure about the suitability of any individual recipes or foodstuffs, please consult a registered dietitian for guidance. (To find a registered dietician in your area, refer to the useful contact numbers provided on pages 206–207.)

BREAKFASTS

Muesli Munch
MAKES 7 CUPS

Vegetarian ◆ Heart Smart ◆ Diabetic

180 g (6 tbsp) honey
500 ml (2 cups) rolled oats, uncooked
250 ml (1 cup) wheat germ
250 ml (1 cup) bran cereal
125 ml (½ cup) mixed nuts, chopped
125 ml (½ cup) sunflower seeds
250 ml (1 cup) dried fruit, chopped
250 ml (1 cup) raisins
62 ml (¼ cup) skimmed milk powder

Melt the honey in a saucepan with a little water (about 2 tbsp). Add all the remaining ingredients, mix well and remove from heat. Spread the mixture on a baking sheet and bake in a cool oven at 160 °C for 25 minutes. Allow to cool and store in an airtight container. Serve with fat-free yoghurt, buttermilk, fruit juice or skimmed milk.

NUTRITIONAL INFORMATION PER PORTION			
Fat (g)	Carbohydrate (g)	Protein (g)	Energy (Cal)
5	31	5	179

Quick & Convenient Alternatives
Refer to the muesli listings in the Shopping Lists on pages 31–33 for a range of alternatives.

Cheesy Haddock Bake

SERVES 4

Heart Smart ◆ Diabetic

2 large haddock fillets (about 225 g), skinned, deboned and flaked
250 g (1 cup) fat-free chunky cottage cheese with chives
125 g (½ punnet) mushrooms, chopped
1 small onion, chopped
10 ml (2 tsp) lemon juice
5 ml (1 tsp) freshly chopped fennel or dill
a pinch each of nutmeg, salt and pepper
1 egg, lightly beaten

Conventional oven: Mix the haddock, cottage cheese, mushrooms and onion together. Add the lemon juice, herbs, seasoning and egg. Scoop equal amounts into four small, ovenproof dishes (or use one large serving dish) and cover with foil. Stand the dishes in a roasting pan containing enough water to come halfway up the sides of the dishes. Bake at 180 °C for 20 minutes until the mixture has set. Serve hot with whole-wheat toast.

Microwave oven: Mix the haddock, cottage cheese, mushrooms and onion together. Add the lemon juice, herbs, seasoning and egg. Scoop equal amounts into four small, ovenproof dishes (or use one large serving dish) and cover with clingwrap. Stand the dishes in a container with enough water to reach halfway up the sides of the dishes. Cook on full (100%) power for 10–12 minutes, until the mixture has set. Serve hot with whole-wheat toast.

NUTRITIONAL INFORMATION PER PORTION			
Fat	Carbohydrate	Protein	Energy
(g)	(g)	(g)	(Cal)
3	4	24	141

Quick & Convenient Alternatives
Pick 'n Pay Choice Haddock Mornay – frozen
Pick 'n Pay Choice Smoked Haddock in Rich Cheese Sauce – frozen

Creamy Ricotta Bake

SERVES 3

Vegetarian ◆ Heart Smart ◆ Diabetic

200 g ricotta cheese
1 egg-white, beaten until stiff
1–2 fresh chillies, chopped
3 ml (½ tsp) nutmeg
5 ml (1 tsp) fresh chives, chopped
salt and pepper to taste

Combine the cheese and the beaten egg-white. Add the chilli, herbs and seasoning. Pour into a soufflé dish prepared with Spray and Cook. Bake at 180°C for 20–30 minutes. Top with chopped peppadews, sun-dried tomatoes or olives, and serve with fresh seed loaf or crusty bread.

NUTRITIONAL INFORMATION PER PORTION			
Fat (g)	Carbohydrate (g)	Protein (g)	Energy (Cal)
5	4	9	98

Spanish Omelette

SERVES 1–2

Vegetarian ◆ Heart Smart ◆ Diabetic

half an onion, peeled and chopped
4–6 mushrooms, sliced
1 gherkin, chopped or sliced
1 small tomato, chopped
2–3 fresh basil leaves, chopped
salt and pepper to taste
2 eggs, beaten together with a little milk
60 g (3 tbsp) fat-free cottage cheese, plain or flavoured

Lightly cook the onion, mushrooms and gherkin in a little stock or water. Add the tomato and basil and season to taste. Mix the beaten egg and the cottage cheese together until smooth. Add to the pan containing the other ingredients and allow the egg to cook through without stirring, carefully lifting sections of the omelette from the bottom of the pan with a spatula. Serve for breakfast or as a main meal.

NUTRITIONAL INFORMATION PER PORTION			
Fat (g)	Carbohydrate (g)	Protein (g)	Energy (Cal)
6	7	12	123

Eggs Benedict
SERVES 1–2

Vegetarian ◆ Diabetic ◆ Microwave

FOR THE SAVOURY SAUCE
3 ml (½ tsp) salt
a pinch of cayenne pepper
5 ml (1 tsp) prepared English mustard
12 ml (1 tbsp) cornflour
12 ml (1 tbsp) cheese powder
125 ml (½ cup) skimmed milk

FOR THE CRUST AND FILLING
2 eggs, poached
2 English muffins/crumpets, lightly toasted
2 slices lean, cooked ham

Conventional oven: Prepare the sauce by mixing the salt, pepper, mustard, cornflour and cheese powder to a paste with a little milk. Bring the remaining milk to the boil, then allow to simmer for 5 minutes. Add to the cornflour paste, and return to the heat. Stir continuously until the mixture thickens, then remove from the heat. Poach the eggs to the desired degree and set aside, keeping them warm. Lightly toast the muffins/crumpets and set aside, keeping them warm. Now place a slice of ham on each toasted muffin/crumpet, and then a poached egg on top of the ham. Top with the savoury sauce and serve immediately.

Microwave oven: Prepare the sauce by mixing the salt, pepper, mustard, cornflour and cheese powder to a paste with a little milk. Bring the remaining milk to the boil in a microwave jug by cooking on full (100%) power for about 2 minutes. Add the cornflour paste and stir well. Cook for a further 1–2 minutes, stirring intermittently, until the mixture is thick and smooth, then set it aside. Meanwhile, poach the eggs to desired degree. Warm the muffins/crumpets in the microwave for a few seconds. Now place a slice of ham on each toasted muffin/crumpet, and then a poached egg on top of the ham. Top with the savoury sauce and serve immediately.

NUTRITIONAL INFORMATION PER PORTION			
Fat (g)	Carbohydrate (g)	Protein (g)	Energy (Cal)
10	32	21	328

Quick & Convenient Alternatives
Woolworths English Muffins
Pick 'n Pay Foodhall British Crumpets
Royco Cheddar Cheese Sauce – packet
Pick 'n Pay Choice Cheese Sauce – ready-made
Walnut Ridge Creamy Cheese Mmm ... Fresh Sauce – ready-made

CHEF'S TIP
For the Eggs Benedict, you may want to use 60 ml (¼ cup) grated, mature Cheddar cheese instead of the cheese powder. Add the grated cheese to the thickened, cooked sauce.

Scrambled Egg with Salmon
SERVES 2–4

Heart Smart ◆ Diabetic

4 eggs, separated
3 ml (½ tsp) baking powder
60 ml (¼ cup) fat-free, smooth cottage cheese
(savoury flavour if desired)
3 ml (½ tsp) salt
a pinch of black pepper or cayenne pepper
5 ml (1 tsp) fresh chives, chopped
125 g smoked salmon, cut into small strips

Whisk the egg-whites until foamy, then add the baking powder. Meanwhile mix the yolks, cottage cheese, salt and pepper together. Now add the beaten egg-whites to the yolk mixture and mix to a uniform texture. Pour into a heated, non-stick pan, or a pan prepared with Spray and Cook, and allow to cook slowly. Draw liquid egg from the edge of the pan to the centre using a spatula, until all the egg is cooked, yet moist. Sprinkle with chopped chives and salmon strips. Serve immediately with hot toast and grilled tomatoes.

NUTRITIONAL INFORMATION PER PORTION			
Fat (g)	Carbohydrate (g)	Protein (g)	Energy (Cal)
10	1	18	206

DIETICIAN'S TIP
If you suffer from high blood cholesterol, substitute half the number of egg-yolks with egg-whites.

Zippy Breakfast Shakes
SERVES 2

Vegetarian ◆ Heart Smart ◆ Diabetic

MIXED FRUIT SHAKE
half a pineapple, peeled and cubed
2 bananas, peeled and sliced
5 ml (1 tsp) lemon juice
175 ml (1 small tub) fat-free strawberry yoghurt
4 ice blocks

APRICOT CREAM
180 ml (¾ cup) apricot juice
125 ml (½ cup) fat-free plain yoghurt
62 ml (¼ cup) pineapple juice

COFFEE DREAM
250 ml (1 cup) skimmed milk
5 ml (1 tsp) instant coffee
5 ml (1 tsp) vanilla essence
a pinch of cinnamon

MANGO SWIRL
125 ml (½ cup) fresh mango pulp
125 ml (½ cup) orange juice
125 ml (½ cup) buttermilk or fat-free plain yoghurt

NUTRITIONAL INFORMATION PER PORTION				
Flavour	**Fat** (g)	**Carbohydrate** (g)	**Protein** (g)	**Energy** (Cal)
Mixed Fruit	1	34	5	158
Apricot Cream	Trace	16	2	82
Coffee Dream	Trace	6	5	43
Mango Swirl	1	25	3	113

Mix all the ingredients for your chosen shake together thoroughly. Blend in a liquidizer until smooth. Serve chilled.

Flapjacks
SERVES 4–6

Vegetarian ◆ Heart Smart ◆ Diabetic

1 egg
30 ml (2 tbsp) castor sugar
5 ml (1 tsp) vanilla essence
250 ml (1 cup) cake flour
10 ml (2 tsp) baking powder
a pinch of salt
180 ml (¾ cup) skimmed milk

Whisk together the egg, castor sugar and vanilla. Sift the dry ingredients together. Add this to the egg mixture alternately with the milk. Beat until a smooth, thin batter is formed. Refrigerate for 30 minutes. Drop spoonfuls of batter onto a hot, non-stick pan or a pan prepared with Spray and Cook. Once browned on the one side and bubbles form on the top surface, flip the flapjack over to brown the other side. Serve hot with syrup.

NUTRITIONAL INFORMATION PER PORTION			
Fat (g)	Carbohydrate (g)	Protein (g)	Energy (Cal)
1	29	5	152

Quick & Convenient Alternatives
Pillsbury Crumpet/Waffle Mix – packet
Wheaton's Brumpets – packet

PATÉS, DIPS & STARTERS

Smoked Angelfish Paté
SERVES 4–6

Heart Smart ◆ Diabetic

1 small smoked angelfish, flaked
250 g (1 tub) fat-free smooth cottage cheese
5 ml (1 tsp) lemon juice
5 ml (1 tsp) hot English mustard
15 ml (1 tbsp) fresh chives, chopped
30 g (1 heaped tbsp) Trim Mayonnaise
salt and pepper to taste

Blend all the ingredients together until smooth. Serve chilled with rice cakes, melba toast, wafers or crudités.

NUTRITIONAL INFORMATION PER PORTION			
Fat (g)	Carbohydrate (g)	Protein (g)	Energy (Cal)
2	2	12	74

CHEF'S TIP
This paté is best when made a day in advance. It is also suitable for freezing.

Microwave Chicken Liver Paté

SERVES 10–12

Diabetic ◆ Microwave

250 g chicken livers, cleaned and dried
1 small onion, chopped
40 g (½ cup) mushrooms, chopped
1 bay leaf
1 sprig fresh thyme, finely chopped
3 ml (a large pinch) salt
black pepper to taste
125 ml (½ cup) skimmed milk
60 ml (¼ cup) brandy/port/orange juice
150 g (1 cup) fat-free cottage cheese

Combine the livers, onion and mushroom, and add the bay leaf, thyme, salt and pepper. Cook the mixture in the milk on full (100%) power for 4–6 minutes, until the livers are done. Remove the bay leaf and purée the mixture in a blender. Add the brandy/port/orange juice and cheese, and blend until a smooth texture is obtained. Scoop into individual serving bowls or one large bowl as desired and allow the paté to cool overnight.

NUTRITIONAL INFORMATION PER PORTION			
Fat (g)	Carbohydrate (g)	Protein (g)	Energy (Cal)
1	2	8	59

DIETICIAN'S TIP
Organ meats, while being unsuitable for those with high blood cholesterol, are a good source of iron for those with iron-deficiency anaemia.

Guacamole

SERVES 6–8

(MAKES ABOUT 250 g)

Vegetarian ◆ Heart Smart ◆ Diabetic

1 ripe medium avocado (about 230 g)
15 g (1 tbsp) onion, grated
1 small clove garlic, crushed
10 ml (2 tsp) lemon juice
salt, black pepper and cayenne pepper to taste
a splash each of Tabasco and
Worcestershire Sauce

Cut the avocado in half and remove the stone and skin. Combine with all the other ingredients and blend until smooth. Chill for about 30 minutes. Serve on a bed of lettuce with crudités or tortillas.

NUTRITIONAL INFORMATION PER PORTION			
Fat (g)	Carbohydrate (g)	Protein (g)	Energy (Cal)
5	2	1	53

Mexican Salsa

SERVES 4–6

Vegetarian ◆ Heart Smart ◆ Diabetic

1 ripe tomato, finely chopped
1 small onion, finely chopped
30 ml (2 tbsp) freshly chopped coriander leaves
1 fresh chilli, finely minced
125 ml (½ cup) whole kernel corn
salt and pepper to taste

Mix all the ingredients together. Season to taste and chill. Serve with crudités, bread sticks or tortillas.

NUTRITIONAL INFORMATION PER PORTION			
Fat (g)	Carbohydrate (g)	Protein (g)	Energy (Cal)
trace	5	1	28

Quick & Convenient Alternatives
Pick 'n Pay Foodhall Mexican Dip Selection – fresh
Crosse & Blackwell Salsa Sauce – bottle
Old El Paso Salsa – bottle

Hummus
SERVES 4–6

Vegetarian ◆ Heart Smart ◆ Diabetic

120 g (½ cup) chickpeas, cooked or tinned and drained
15 ml (1 tbsp) fat-free plain yoghurt
1 clove garlic, crushed
a pinch each of black pepper, cayenne pepper and salt
15 ml (1 tbsp) lemon juice
5 ml (1 tsp) freshly chopped coriander
10 ml (2 tsp) toasted sesame seeds (optional)

Blend all the ingredients in a liquidizer until smooth. Chill and serve with melba toast or French loaf.

NUTRITIONAL INFORMATION PER PORTION			
Fat (g)	Carbohydrate (g)	Protein (g)	Energy (Cal)
1	6	2	43

SOUPS

Italian Bean Soup

SERVES 4–6

Vegetarian ◆ Heart Smart ◆ Diabetic

2 large carrots, peeled and sliced
1 clove garlic, crushed
1 large onion or 2 medium onions, peeled and chopped
2 sticks celery, sliced
2 courgettes, topped and tailed and sliced
2 medium potatoes, peeled and sliced
a large wedge of cabbage (about 300 g), finely shredded
1 250 ml (5 cups) vegetable stock
6–8 large ripe tomatoes, skinned and chopped or
2 x 410-g cans whole peeled tomatoes, chopped
200 g (1 cup) cooked beans
(e.g. butter beans, haricot beans, cannellini beans etc.)
salt and pepper to taste

Place all the prepared vegetables, except the tomatoes and beans, in a large saucepan. Add the stock and bring to the boil. Reduce the heat and simmer, covered, for 1½–2 hours or until the soup has thickened. During the last 15 minutes of cooking time, stir in the drained, cooked beans and the tomato. Season to taste and garnish with chopped parsley.

NUTRITIONAL INFORMATION PER PORTION			
Fat (g)	Carbohydrate (g)	Protein (g)	Energy (Cal)
1	40	10	242

Quick & Convenient Alternatives
Tuscan Bean & Pasta Dining-In-Soup – ready-made
Woolworths Italian Bean & Tomato Soup – fresh

Sweet Potato & Ginger Soup

SERVES 6–8

Heart Smart ◆ Diabetic

1 orange, juice and grated rind
5 ml (1 tsp) curry powder
⅓ cup freshly chopped coriander leaves
5 ml (1 tsp) sugar
30 ml (2 tbsp) freshly grated ginger
3 large sweet potatoes (about 1 kg),
peeled and cut into chunks
4 parsnips, peeled and diced
3 large leeks, thinly sliced
2 large carrots, thinly sliced
10 ml (2 tsp) salt
1 litre (4 cups) chicken stock
500 ml (2 cups) skimmed milk
fresh coriander leaves to garnish
pepper to taste

Mix together the orange juice and rind, the curry powder, coriander, sugar, ginger, sweet potato, parsnips, leeks, carrots and 2–3 tbsp stock, and cook over moderate heat for about 6 minutes. Add the seasoning, the remainder of the stock and the milk and simmer, covered, for about 30 minutes or until all the vegetables are tender. Blend to a pulp in a food processor, and reheat if necessary. Garnish with fresh coriander leaves. Serve hot with toasted bagels.

NUTRITIONAL INFORMATION PER PORTION			
Fat (g)	Carbohydrate (g)	Protein (g)	Energy (Cal)
1	44	6	228

Chilled Summer Soup

SERVES 3–4

Vegetarian ◆ Heart Smart ◆ Diabetic

280 ml (1¼ cup) fat-free plain yoghurt
280 ml (1¼ cup) tomato juice
half an orange, juice and grated rind
a slice of cucumber, 2.5 cm thick and finely chopped
1 red or yellow pepper, seeded and chopped
salt and pepper to taste

Whisk the yoghurt and the tomato juice together. Add the remaining ingredients and liquidize. Season to taste and chill. Serve with crusty baguettes or whole-wheat rolls

NUTRITIONAL INFORMATION PER PORTION			
Fat (g)	Carbohydrate (g)	Protein (g)	Energy (Cal)
trace	13	6	79

Carrot & Coriander Soup
SERVES 4–6

Vegetarian ◆ Heart Smart ◆ Diabetic

2 cubes stock
1 litre (4 cups) boiling water
5 ml (1 tsp) crushed garlic (about 3 cloves)
1 onion, peeled and chopped
5 ml (1 tsp) crushed ginger, or
about 4 cm fresh root ginger, peeled and grated
1 kg carrots, topped and tailed and cut into rings
125 ml (½ cup) freshly chopped coriander leaves

Dissolve the stock cubes in the boiling water. Brown the garlic, onion and ginger in a little (about 2–3 tbsp) stock for 6–8 minutes. Add the carrots and the remaining stock and cook until the carrots are tender. Add the coriander about 5 minutes before the end of cooking time. Remove from heat and liquidize in a food processor until smooth. Garnish with fresh coriander leaves. Serve hot or cold with fresh, crusty bread.

NUTRITIONAL INFORMATION PER PORTION			
Fat	**Carbohydrate**	**Protein**	**Energy**
(g)	(g)	(g)	(Cal)
trace	15	2	90

Quick & Convenient Alternatives
Woolworths Carrot & Coriander Soup – fresh
Baxter's Healthy Choice Carrot, Onion & Chickpea Soup – canned

> ### DIETICIAN'S TIP
> *All orange fruits and vegetables are excellent sources of beta-carotene, which has anti-cancer and other health properties.*

Curried Cauliflower Soup

SERVES 4

Heart Smart ◆ Diabetic

2 onions, peeled and finely chopped
500 ml (2 cups) chicken stock
2 ml (½ tsp) curry powder
1 cauliflower (leaves trimmed), broken into florets
75 ml (4–5 tbsp) flour
500 ml (2 cups) skimmed milk
2 bay leaves
salt and pepper to taste

Cook the onions in a little stock, adding the curry powder. Add the cauliflower and cook for 5 minutes. Add the flour, and cook for a further 5 minutes. Add the remaining ingredients and allow to simmer for about 30 minutes. Remove the bay leaves, and blend the mixture in a liquidizer until smooth. Serve hot, garnished with parsley and croûtons.

NUTRITIONAL INFORMATION PER PORTION			
Fat	**Carbohydrate**	**Protein**	**Energy**
(g)	(g)	(g)	(Cal)
1	20	8	126

Haddock & Corn Chowder

SERVES 8

Heart Smart ◆ Diabetic

3 rashers back bacon (fat trimmed), chopped
2 medium onions, peeled and chopped
30 ml (2 tbsp) cake flour
375 ml (1½ cups) chicken stock
375 ml (1½ cups) water
6 large potatoes (about 900 g), cut into small cubes
2 stalks celery, chopped
300 g (2 cups) green beans, cut into 3-cm pieces
300 g (2 cups) frozen corn
250 ml (1 cup) skimmed milk
3 large smoked haddock fillets (about 500 g), flaked
10 ml (2 tsp) Worcestershire sauce
a pinch of nutmeg
salt and pepper to taste
45 ml (3 tbsp) freshly chopped dill or parsley

Cook the chopped bacon until crisp, then set it aside on absorbent paper. Cook the onion until soft, then stir in the flour. Add the stock and the water and bring to the boil. Add the potatoes and the celery and simmer, covered, for 10 minutes. Add the green beans and the corn and cook for 5 minutes. Stir in the milk, the fish, the Worcestershire sauce, nutmeg and seasoning. Simmer gently until the fish is cooked and the potatoes are soft. Stir in the parsley and garnish with bacon bits. Serve with fresh, crusty bread.

NUTRITIONAL INFORMATION PER PORTION			
Fat	Carbohydrate	Protein	Energy
(g)	(g)	(g)	(Cal)
2	38	23	273

Red Pepper & Basil Soup

SERVES 4

Vegetarian ◆ Heart Smart ◆ Diabetic

3 red peppers, seeded and chopped
1 large onion, chopped
1 clove garlic, crushed
625 ml (2½ cups) vegetable stock
30 ml (2 tbsp) tomato paste
2 carrots, chopped
1 potato, peeled and cubed
1 large bunch fresh basil, chopped
250 ml (1 cup) skimmed milk
5 ml (1 tsp) sugar
5 ml (1 tsp) paprika
2 ml (a pinch) salt
black pepper
fat-free plain yoghurt and
grated orange rind to garnish

Cook the peppers, onion and garlic in a little of the vegetable stock for 4–5 minutes until tender. Add the remaining stock, and the tomato paste, carrots and potato. Bring to the boil, cover and simmer for 20 minutes. Add the basil, milk, sugar and seasoning 5 minutes before the end of the cooking time. Purée the soup in a liquidizer, reheat and season to taste. Garnish with a swirl of yoghurt and grated orange rind. Serve with toasted ciabatta bread or crispy rolls.

NUTRITIONAL INFORMATION PER PORTION			
Fat (g)	Carbohydrate (g)	Protein (g)	Energy (Cal)
1	18	4	99

Quick & Convenient Alternative
Baxters Italian Tomato with Basil Soup – can

Orange, Mango & Butternut Soup

SERVES 4–6

Heart Smart ◆ Diabetic ◆ Microwave

2 cloves garlic, peeled and crushed
1 small onion, peeled and finely chopped
2 large butternuts (about 600 g),
peeled and cut into chunks
1 litre (4 cups) chicken stock
250 ml (1 cup) orange juice
3 ml (½ tsp) ground nutmeg
1 ripe mango, peeled and chopped
salt and pepper to taste
5 ml (1 tsp) curry powder (optional)

Place the garlic, onion, butternut and half the stock into a covered microwave dish. Cook on full (100%) power for 5–7 minutes until the butternut is tender. Add the remaining stock and orange juice and cook for a further 2–3 minutes. Add the nutmeg and the mango and season to taste. Blend to a smooth consistency in a liquidizer. Serve hot or cold with fresh ciabatta bread.

NUTRITIONAL INFORMATION PER PORTION			
Fat	Carbohydrate	Protein	Energy
(g)	(g)	(g)	(Cal)
1	25	2	119

Quick & Convenient Alternatives
Pick 'n Pay Choice Butternut Soup – ready-made
Pick 'n Pay Foodhall Butternut Soup Pack – fresh

Creamy Broccoli Soup

SERVES 6–8

Vegetarian ◆ Heart Smart ◆ Diabetic

2 onions, chopped
4 cubes vegetable stock, dissolved in
1½ litres boiling water/rooibos tea
125 ml (½ cup) cake flour
3 large stalks fresh broccoli,
broken into florets (about 750 g)
1 large tomato, chopped
2 ml (a pinch) each of thyme, rosemary and nutmeg
salt and pepper to taste
250 ml (1 cup) skimmed milk
200 ml (¾ cup) fat-free plain yoghurt

Cook the onions in a small amount of stock, until tender. Stir in the flour and cook for a minute to form a smooth paste. Add the rest of the stock gradually, stirring continuously. Add the broccoli, tomato, herbs and seasoning. Bring to the boil and simmer, while covered, until the broccoli is tender. Allow to cool slightly, then blend in a liquidizer. Add the milk and the yoghurt and heat through – DO NOT BOIL. Serve hot or chilled with toasted seed loaf.

NUTRITIONAL INFORMATION PER PORTION			
Fat (g)	Carbohydrate (g)	Protein (g)	Energy (Cal)
1	16	7	103

DIETICIAN'S TIP
It is now believed that broccoli is one of the top eight cancer-fighting foods·

SALADS AND VEGETABLES

Grilled Vegetables with Soft Herbed Cheese
SERVES 6–8

Vegetarian ◆ Heart Smart ◆ Diabetic

half a large butternut (about 150–200 g),
peeled and cut into chunks
90 ml (6 tbsp) balsamic vinegar
1 clove garlic, crushed
125 ml (½ cup) vegetable stock
2 tbsp honey
2 courgettes, cut into 3-cm chunks
4–6 patty pans, cut into quarters
250 g baby vegetables of your choice
16 cherry tomatoes
16 button mushrooms, cleaned
8 black olives, pitted
150 g (1 cup) goat's milk cheese or ricotta cheese
30 ml (2 tbsp) each of freshly chopped basil and coriander
salt and black pepper to taste

Steam the butternut until it is cooked but firm, then set it aside. Mix the balsamic vinegar, garlic, stock and honey together. Mix together all the vegetables and olives, and drizzle with the honey mixture. Arrange the vegetables in an ovenproof dish and cover with foil. Bake at 200 °C for 15–20 minutes, ensuring that you turn the vegetables frequently. Meanwhile, cut the cheese into small blocks and roll each block in the fresh herbs. Arrange the vegetables in a large serving dish, season, add cheese blocks and drizzle with additional balsamic vinegar if desired.

NUTRITIONAL INFORMATION PER PORTION			
Fat (g)	Carbohydrate (g)	Protein (g)	Energy (Cal)
3	19	5	125

Quick & Convenient Alternative
Woolworths Char-Grilled Roast Vegetables

Potato & Broccoli Frittata
SERVES 6–8

Vegetarian ◆ Heart Smart ◆ Diabetic

500 g baby potatoes, whole and unpeeled
300 g (1 punnet) fresh broccoli
4 eggs, beaten
60 ml (¼ cup) fat-free cottage cheese
125 ml (½ cup) skimmed milk
1 x 210 g can sweetcorn
seasoning to taste

Cook the potatoes in lightly salted water until they are soft, but firm. Allow to cool and slice each potato in half. Steam the broccoli until tender. Combine all the ingredients and mix thoroughly. Using a non-stick pan, cook the mixture over a low heat for 15 minutes (until the egg is cooked through), then place under the grill for about 5 minutes until golden brown. Serve immediately.

NUTRITIONAL INFORMATION PER PORTION			
Fat (g)	Carbohydrate (g)	Protein (g)	Energy (Cal)
4	20	9	154

Medley of Fruity Sweet Potato with Nuts
SERVES 6–8

Vegetarian ◆ Heart Smart ◆ Diabetic

1 large onion, peeled and chopped
3 large sweet potatoes, peeled and chopped
170 ml (⅔ cup) stock
15 ml (2 tbsp) sultanas
1 clove garlic, peeled and crushed
1 x 2-cm piece root ginger, peeled and finely grated
1 orange, juice and grated rind
2 ml (½ tsp) ground cinnamon (optional)
45 ml (3 tbsp) toasted pumpkin seeds or nuts of your choice

Cook the onion and the sweet potato in the stock over low heat for about 8 minutes. Add the sultanas, garlic, ginger, orange juice and rind. Bring to the boil, then cover and simmer for 25 minutes or until the sweet potato is tender. Sprinkle with nuts and cinnamon just before serving. Serve as a vegetable accompaniment.

NUTRITIONAL INFORMATION PER PORTION			
Fat (g)	Carbohydrate (g)	Protein (g)	Energy (Cal)
1	39	4	204

DIETICIAN'S TIP
Although both nuts and seeds are high in fat, the fats are of a healthy, unsaturated type.

Roast Courgette & Butternut Salad

SERVES 6

Vegetarian ◆ Heart Smart ◆ Diabetic

FOR THE SALAD
14 baby potatoes, halved
1 medium butternut, peeled, seeded and cut into chunks
5 medium courgettes, trimmed and sliced
15 ml (1 tbsp) freshly chopped marjoram
15 ml (1 tbsp) toasted sunflower seeds
salt and pepper to taste

FOR THE DRESSING
5 ml (1 tsp) sugar
1 clove garlic, peeled and crushed
3 ml (½ tsp) mustard powder
60 ml (¼ cup) balsamic vinegar
5 ml (1 tsp) basil pesto
salt and freshly ground black pepper

Boil the potatoes in lightly salted water until soft, but firm – then set aside. Arrange the chunks of butternut in a roasting pan with a little stock or water. Season with salt and pepper and cook, covered, at 180 °C for 30 minutes. Give the pan a good shake every now and then to prevent the butternut from sticking to the bottom, and add more stock if it is drying out. Add the courgettes and roast, uncovered, for a further 10 minutes. Allow to cool. Add the halved potatoes to the butternut and courgettes. Sprinkle with marjoram and sunflower seeds. Mix together all the ingredients for the dressing, and pour over vegetables. Serve at room temperature on a bed of couscous.

NUTRITIONAL INFORMATION PER PORTION			
Fat (g)	Carbohydrate (g)	Protein (g)	Energy (Cal)
2	9	2	65

Grilled Black Mushrooms

SERVES 6

Vegetarian ◆ Heart Smart ◆ Diabetic ◆ Microwave

6 large black mushrooms
3 ml (½ tsp) salt
1 clove garlic, peeled and crushed
30 ml (3 tbsp) Lite Salad Dressing
freshly ground black pepper
1 tbsp Parmesan cheese (optional)
15 ml (1 tbsp) freshly chopped oreganum

Place the cleaned mushrooms stem side up on a greased baking tray. Mix together the salt, garlic and salad dressing. Using a brush dipped in this mixture, coat the mushrooms evenly. Sprinkle with freshly ground black pepper, oreganum and Parmesan (optional). Grill in a conventional oven for 5–8 minutes, or microwave for 3–5 minutes on full (100%) power. Serve as a starter or as a vegetable accompaniment.

NUTRITIONAL INFORMATION PER PORTION			
Fat (g)	Carbohydrate (g)	Protein (g)	Energy (Cal)
2	2	1	28

Green Salad with Tangy Mango & Mint Dressing

SERVES 4–6

Vegetarian ◆ Heart Smart ◆ Diabetic

FOR THE SALAD
shredded lettuce leaves or
Chinese cabbage
spring onions
mango slices
green pepper, seeded and cut into strips
cucumber slices

FOR THE DRESSING
1 red chilli, finely chopped
1 ripe mango, peeled and removed from pip
15 ml (1 tbsp) fruit chutney
175 ml (1 small tub) low-fat plain yoghurt
30 ml (2 tbsp) coconut milk
2 tbsp freshly chopped mint leaves
shredded almonds to garnish

To make the salad: Prepare a tossed salad and sprinkle with mango slices. **To make the dressing:** Combine all the ingredients and blend in a food processor until smooth. Drizzle the salad with dressing and garnish with shredded almonds. Serve well chilled, with fresh bread.

NUTRITIONAL INFORMATION PER PORTION			
Fat (g)	Carbohydrate (g)	Protein (g)	Energy (Cal)
1	23	3	114

Spicy Carrot Salad

SERVES 6–8

Vegetarian ◆ Heart Smart ◆ Diabetic

500 g baby carrots
1 medium green pepper, seeded and cut into rings
1 medium onion, peeled and cut into rings
1 x 82-g packet Maggi Tomato Soup
250 ml (1 cup) water
180 ml (⅔ cup) white vinegar
250 ml (1 cup) sugar
10 ml (2 tsp) Worcestershire Sauce
5 ml (1 tsp) mustard powder
salt and pepper to taste
pineapple pieces (optional)

Steam or microwave the carrots until they are cooked, but firm. Layer the carrots, green peppers and onions in a deep casserole dish with a lid, and set aside. Mix all other ingredients together in a saucepan and bring to the boil, stirring continuously. Boil for 2 minutes. Pour the hot sauce over the vegetables (and the pineapple, if included). Cover and allow to cool in a refrigerator. Leave the vegetables to marinate for two days before use. Serve chilled.

NUTRITIONAL INFORMATION PER PORTION			
Fat	**Carbohydrate**	**Protein**	**Energy**
(g)	(g)	(g)	(Cal)
trace	35	1	151

Mexican Tuna Salad

SERVES 4

Heart Smart ◆ Diabetic

250 g pasta of your choice
1 x 185-g can tuna in brine, drained
45 ml (3 tbsp) sweetcorn kernels
45 ml (3 tbsp) kidney beans, cooked
1 carrot, grated
2 tomatoes, cut into wedges
30 ml (2 tbsp) Trim mayonnaise
60 ml (¼ cup) fat-free salad dressing
60 ml (¼ cup) skimmed milk
salt and pepper to taste
half a chilli, minced
1 small head of lettuce

Cook the pasta according to the manufacturer's instructions. Drain and set aside. Mix all the ingredients together lightly, with the exception of the lettuce. Serve on a bed of lettuce, well chilled.

NUTRITIONAL INFORMATION PER PORTION			
Fat	Carbohydrate	Protein	Energy
(g)	(g)	(g)	(Cal)
5	45	22	331

Quick & Convenient Alternatives
Woolworths/Pick 'n Pay Fresh Pasta
Pick 'n Pay Choice Mexican Tuna chunks with Sweetcorn & Kidney Beans
Woolworths/Pick 'n Pay Salad Pack

Thai Chicken Salad

SERVES 4–6

Heart Smart ◆ Diabetic

1 cube chicken or vegetable stock, crumbled
250 ml (1 cup) boiling water
2 chicken breast fillets
30 ml (2 tbsp) uncooked long grain rice
6 spring onions, chopped
1 large tomato, cut into wedges
half an English cucumber, sliced and halved
2 large fresh chillies, chopped
30 ml (2 tbsp) freshly chopped mint
30 ml (2 tbsp) freshly chopped coriander leaves
15 ml (1 tbsp) freshly chopped lemon grass
1 small head of cos or iceberg lettuce
60 ml (¼ cup) lemon juice
15 ml (1 tbsp) Thai fish sauce
15 ml (1 tbsp) sugar

Dissolve the stock cube in the water, and bring to the boil in a saucepan. Add the chicken and allow to simmer, covered, until cooked and tender. Allow the chicken to stand in the stock for 10 minutes before draining. Keep 1–2 tbsp of the stock, and discard the rest. Chop the chicken into bite-sized pieces, and set aside to cool. Place the rice in a dry pan and stir over moderate heat for about 5 minutes or until lightly browned. Grind the rice to a fine powder in a food processor, or use a pestle and mortar. (The rice is not essential in this recipe, but it does add a unique flavour). Combine the chicken, powdered rice, spring onions, tomato, cucumber, chillies, mint, coriander and lemon grass in a bowl. Line a salad bowl with shredded lettuce leaves and spoon the chicken mixture onto this. Mix together the lemon juice, fish sauce, sugar and reserved stock and drizzle this over the salad just before serving.

NUTRITIONAL INFORMATION PER PORTION			
Fat (g)	Carbohydrate (g)	Protein (g)	Energy (Cal)
3	16	14	160

Spicy Hot & Cold Ostrich Salad with Honey-Mustard Dressing
SERVES 4

Heart Smart ◆ Diabetic

1 stock cube
10 ml (2 tsp) salt,
dissolved in a cup of water
juice of a small lemon
15 ml (1 tbsp) mild curry powder
30 ml (2 tbsp) mustard
75 ml (2 heaped tbsp) honey
250 g ostrich meat, cut into strips
fresh green salad of your choice

Mix the stock, salt water, lemon juice, curry powder, mustard and honey together thoroughly, and pour over the meat strips. Cover, and refrigerate for 5–6 hours. Place the meat strips (in the marinade) in a covered baking tray or casserole dish and cook at 180 °C for about an hour – take care not to let the meat dry out. Meanwhile, prepare a fresh green salad. Spoon the hot meat and the sauce over the salad and toss lightly just before serving. The hot meat tends to wilt lettuce leaves, so add the meat to the salad just before serving. Serve immediately with crusty bread.

NUTRITIONAL INFORMATION PER PORTION			
Fat (g)	Carbohydrate (g)	Protein (g)	Energy (Cal)
3	29	14	187

Quick & Convenient Alternative
Heinz Honey Dijon Dressing – sachet

DIETICIAN'S TIP
Not only is ostrich meat an extra lean meat – it is also rich in iron and low in cholesterol. Furthermore, ostrich meat currently costs less than other red meat products. Ostrich meat is an ideal substitute for beef or lamb, but it is best served rare to medium-rare. Strong flavours like pepper, mustard and peri-peri best complement the delicate flavour of ostrich meat.

Chilled Cucumber Salad
SERVES 6–8

Vegetarian ◆ Heart Smart ◆ Diabetic

2 cucumbers, grated
1 medium onion, peeled and grated
125 ml (½ cup) fat-free plain yoghurt
10 ml (2 tsp) dill
salt and pepper to taste

Combine all the ingredients, cover and refrigerate. Serve well chilled. This is delicious with lamb kebabs or meatballs.

NUTRITIONAL INFORMATION PER PORTION			
Fat (g)	Carbohydrate (g)	Protein (g)	Energy (Cal)
trace	4	2	30

PASTA

Penne Arrabiatta

SERVES 4

Vegetarian ◆ Heart Smart ◆ Diabetic

1 medium onion, peeled and finely chopped
1 small green pepper, seeded and chopped
2 cloves garlic, crushed
1 x 410-g can tomatoes (or 4 ripe tomatoes), chopped
salt and black pepper to taste
15 ml (1 tbsp) sugar
5 ml (1 tsp) dried basil or 15 ml (1 tbsp) freshly chopped basil
5 ml (1 tsp) chicken or vegetable stock
30 ml (2 tbsp) dry red wine
2–3 chillies, finely chopped or minced
6 black olives (optional)
500 g (1 packet) penne

Place all the ingredients, except the pasta, into a deep saucepan (include the olives if you are using them) and simmer, uncovered, for about 20–30 minutes. Meanwhile, cook the pasta according to the manufacturer's instructions and set it aside, covered, while keeping it warm. Season the sauce to taste and spoon onto a bed of pasta.

NUTRITIONAL INFORMATION PER PORTION			
Fat (g)	Carbohydrate (g)	Protein (g)	Energy (Cal)
2	77	14	407

Quick & Convenient Alternatives
Pick 'n Pay Choice Italian Classic Arrabiatta Sauce – bottle
Pick 'n Pay Choice Italian Classic Chopped Peeled Tomatoes with Chilli

Smoked Salmon Shells
SERVES 4

Heart Smart ◆ Diabetic

500 g large pasta shells
45 ml (3 tbsp) cornflour
a pinch of nutmeg
salt and pepper to taste
500 ml (2 cups) skimmed milk
125 ml (½ cup) chicken stock
150 g smoked salmon, cut into strips
3 tbsp Parmesan cheese
60 ml (¼ cup) freshly chopped basil

Cook the pasta according to the manufacturer's instructions until *al dente*, cover and set aside while keeping it warm. Mix the cornflour, nutmeg, salt and pepper to a smooth paste with a little of the cold milk. Mix the remaining milk with the stock, bring to the boil and add the cornflour paste, stirring until the sauce thickens. Add the salmon strips, half the Parmesan cheese and half the basil to the thickened sauce. Mix lightly and pour over the pasta shells. Garnish with the remaining cheese and basil.

NUTRITIONAL INFORMATION PER PORTION			
Fat (g)	Carbohydrate (g)	Protein (g)	Energy (Cal)
7	77	27	500

CHEF'S TIP
Wild salmon have firm flesh with a delicious flavour – English, Scottish and Irish salmon are particularly good. Farmed salmon are deprived of their natural diet, which commonly causes a less pale flesh. Artificial colourants are added to their feed to ensure a pink flesh.

Chunky Tuna & Broccoli Buttermilk Bake

SERVES 6

Heart Smart ♦ Diabetic

250 g fussili
125 g (½ punnet) mushrooms, cleaned and sliced
1 onion, peeled and chopped
2 cups broccoli florets
5 ml (1 tsp) freshly chopped rosemary needles
30 ml (2 tbsp) soy sauce
3 spring onions, chopped
1 x 185-g can tuna chunks in brine, drained
250 g (1 tub) fat-free smooth cottage cheese
2 eggs
250 ml (1 cup) buttermilk
salt and freshly ground black pepper to taste
2 cloves garlic, peeled and crushed
15 ml (1 tbsp) freshly chopped oreganum
25 g (1 slice) whole-wheat bread,
crusts removed and coarsely grated
5 ml (1 tsp) dried Parmesan cheese (optional)

Cook the pasta in boiling water for 5 minutes, drain and set aside while keeping it warm. Cook the mushrooms, onion, broccoli and rosemary in 2 tbsp water until the mushrooms are soft and the onion is translucent, then add the soy sauce. In a large bowl, mix the spring onions, tuna and cottage cheese. Now beat the eggs and buttermilk together with the salt and pepper. Now combine the broccoli mixture, the tuna mixture and the buttermilk mixture and add the fussili. Spoon into a casserole dish prepared with Spray and Cook. Mix together the garlic, oreganum, bread-crumbs and Parmesan (if used). Sprinkle this over the pasta mixture. Finally, bake at 160 °C for 45 minutes. Leave to settle for 10 minutes once the oven has been switched off. Serve with lightly grilled tomatoes.

NUTRITIONAL INFORMATION PER PORTION			
Fat	Carbohydrate	Protein	Energy
(g)	(g)	(g)	(Cal)
4	30	23	259

Oriental Noodles with Smoked Mussels
SERVES 4

Heart Smart ◆ Diabetic

500 g spaghetti
225 g baby corn, halved lengthways
1 green pepper, seeded and cut into strips
1 bunch spring onions, sliced
2.5 cm fresh root ginger, peeled and grated
1 clove garlic, peeled and crushed
6 tbsp (⅓ cup) orange juice
10 ml (2 tsp) cornflour
60 ml (4 tbsp) dark soy sauce
30 ml (2 tbsp) dry white wine
30 ml (2 tbsp) tomato paste
1 x 105-g can smoked mussels, drained
5 ml (1 tsp) freshly chopped coriander

Cook the pasta according to the manufacturer's instructions, cover and set aside while keeping it warm. Cook the corn, green pepper, spring onions, ginger and garlic in the orange juice for 3–4 minutes. Mix the cornflour to a paste with a little water, then add the soy sauce, wine, tomato paste and half a cup of water. Add this mixture to the vegetables and continue to cook for a further 2–3 minutes, until the sauce thickens. Add the mussels and allow to heat through. Serve on a bed of spaghetti, sprinkled with fresh coriander.

NUTRITIONAL INFORMATION PER PORTION			
Fat (g)	Carbohydrate (g)	Protein (g)	Energy (Cal)
4	90	28	532

Quick & Convenient Alternatives

Woolworths/Pick 'n Pay Fresh Pasta
Royco Sweet 'n Sour Sauce – packet
Woolworths Fresh Smoked Mussels – fresh
Woolworths Sweet 'n Spicy Grill & Bake Sauce – ready-made
Woolworths Oriental Sweet 'n Sour Cook-in-Sauce – can

CHEF'S TIP
The mussels, above, can be replaced with any seafood of your choice.

Creamy Alfredo
SERVES 4–5

Heart Smart ◆ Diabetic

500 g (1 packet) tagliatelle
250 g lean bacon or lean smoked ham, cut into strips
2 cloves garlic, peeled and crushed
30 ml (2 tbsp) dry white wine
250 g (1 punnet) mushrooms, cleaned and sliced
500 ml (2 cups) skimmed milk
2–3 heaped tsp cornflour
2 heaped tsp mushroom stock powder
freshly chopped oreganum to taste

Cook the tagliatelle according to the manufacturer's instructions. Set it aside, covered, and keep it warm. Briefly cook the bacon/ham, garlic and wine in a non-stick frying pan. Add the sliced mushrooms and cook for a further 5 minutes. Add 1½ cups of milk to the bacon and mushroom mixture, and bring to the boil. Mix the cornflour and the stock powder with the remaining milk to form a smooth paste, and add this to the bacon and mushroom mixture. Stir continuously until the sauce thickens. Add the oreganum and serve immediately on a bed of pasta.

NUTRITIONAL INFORMATION PER PORTION			
Fat (g)	Carbohydrate (g)	Protein (g)	Energy (Cal)
4	63	24	410

Quick & Convenient Alternatives
Woolworths/Pick 'n Pay Fresh Pasta
Woolworths Mushroom & White Wine Cook-in Sauce – can
Pick 'n Pay Choice Alfredo Pasta & Sauce – packet
Royco Cheese, Ham & Mushroom Sauce – packet
Royco Alfredo Pasta & Sauce – packet
Napolina Alfredo Pasta & Sauce – packet

DIETICIAN'S TIPS
Remember not to eat meat more than three times per week, and then opt for more fish, chicken, ostrich or game. Avoid smoked foods if you are at risk of cancer.

Chicken Tagliatelle in a Creamy Wine Sauce

SERVES 4

Heart Smart ◆ Diabetic

1 onion, peeled and sliced
2 cloves garlic, peeled and crushed
250 ml (1 cup) white wine
4 skinless chicken fillets, sliced into small pieces
500 g tagliatelle
125 ml (½ cup) skimmed milk
30 ml (2 tbsp) cornflour
5 ml (1 tsp) mustard powder
5 ml (1 tsp) stock powder
125 g (½ punnet) mushrooms
125 g (½ punnet) broccoli

Cook the onion and garlic in a little wine until soft. Add the chicken pieces and allow to brown. Reduce heat and keep warm. Meanwhile, prepare the pasta according to the manufacturer's instructions until *al dente* and set aside. To make the cheese sauce, mix the cornflour, mustard powder and stock powder to a smooth paste with a little milk. Bring the remaining milk to the boil and add a bit to the paste, then add this to the boiling milk again. Add the remaining wine and pour over the chicken mixture. Simmer for 5 minutes, then add the mushrooms and broccoli. Cook for a further 10–15 minutes. Serve on a bed of tagliatelle.

NUTRITIONAL INFORMATION PER PORTION			
Fat (g)	Carbohydrate (g)	Protein (g)	Energy (Cal)
8	75	37	581

Quick & Convenient Alternatives

Woolworths/Pick 'n Pay Fresh Pasta
All Gold Creamy White Wine Cook-in-Sauce – can
Woolworths Char-Grilled Chicken Pasta – fresh
Woolworths Mushroom & White Wine Cook-in-Sauce – can

Ostrich & Lentil Lasagne

SERVES 4

Heart Smart ◆ Diabetic

105 g (½ cup) uncooked brown lentils, or
180 g (1 cup) cooked brown lentils
225 g ostrich mince
1 large onion, chopped
1 stick celery, sliced
1 clove garlic, crushed
a little stock, wine or sherry
5 ml (1 tsp) stock powder
5 ml (1 tsp) dried basil, or
15 ml (3 tsp) freshly chopped basil
5 ml (1 tsp) dried oreganum, or
15 ml (3 tsp) freshly chopped oreganum
5 ml (1 tsp) sugar
1 x 410-g can tomatoes, chopped
30 ml (2 tbsp) tomato paste
2 courgettes, chopped
1 carrot, grated
6 sheets lasagne
125 g (½ tub) fat-free cottage cheese
2 slices whole-wheat bread, crusts removed

Firstly, cook the lentils by adding enough water to cover them, and bring to the boil. Once boiling, reduce the heat and simmer, uncovered, for 20–30 minutes. Check that all the water has been absorbed and that the lentils are tender. Set aside. Now brown the mince, onion, celery and garlic in a saucepan with a little stock, wine or sherry. Add the stock powder, herbs, sugar, tomatoes, tomato paste, courgettes and carrot and simmer for 30 minutes. Add the lentils to the meat mixture, and heat through. Layer the meat, sheets of lasagne and cottage cheese until all the ingredients have been used up, finishing with a layer of cottage cheese. Coarsely grate the bread and sprinkle on top. Cook for a further 30 minutes at 180 °C until golden brown.

NUTRITIONAL INFORMATION PER PORTION			
Fat (g)	Carbohydrate (g)	Protein (g)	Energy (Cal)
4	48	33	458

Quick & Convenient Alternative
Pick 'n Pay Choice Lentils – can

DIETICIAN'S TIP
Lentils and other legumes are an excellent foodstuff for lowering blood cholesterol levels, as well as for stabilizing blood sugar levels.

CHICKEN

Chicken Stroganoff
SERVES 4

Heart Smart ◆ Diabetic

30 ml (2 tbsp) flour
5 ml (1 tsp) paprika
5 ml (1 tsp) dried mixed herbs
salt and black pepper
4–6 chicken breast fillets, cubed
500–750 ml (2–3 cups) chicken stock
1 large onion, chopped
1 clove garlic, crushed
250 g (1 punnet) mushrooms, chopped
80 ml (⅓ cup) dry sherry
80 ml (⅓ cup) fat-free plain yoghurt
10 ml (2 tsp) freshly chopped chives

Mix the flour, paprika, herbs, salt and pepper in a plastic bag and lightly toss in the chicken pieces. Gently cook the seasoned chicken pieces, garlic and onion in a little stock until browned and tender. Add the mushrooms, sherry and remaining stock and cook for a further 10 minutes. Allow the mixture to cook until the sauce is thick and the chicken is cooked. Remove from heat and stir in the yoghurt and chives. Serve with noodles or rice.

NUTRITIONAL INFORMATION PER PORTION			
Fat (g)	Carbohydrate (g)	Protein (g)	Energy (Cal)
10	10	41	317

Quick & Convenient Alternative
Walnut Ridge Creamy Stroganoff Incredible Casserole – ready-made

Thai Green Curry
SERVES 4

Diabetic

750 g chicken breast fillets, cut into cubes
2 small leeks, sliced
250 ml (1 cup) stock
2 fresh chillies, chopped
10 ml (2 tsp) ground coriander
5 ml (1 tsp) cumin
2 ml (½ tsp) nutmeg
10 ml (2 tsp) freshly grated ginger
2 cloves garlic, peeled and crushed
1 lemon, juice and finely grated rind
15 ml (1 tbsp) finely chopped lemon grass
30 ml (2 tbsp) Thai fish sauce
1 x 400-g can coconut milk
25 ml freshly chopped coriander
sesame seeds to garnish

Brown the leeks and the chicken in a little stock for 8–10 minutes. Add all the remaining ingredients except the sesame seeds, and cook for a further 10 minutes. Reduce heat and allow to simmer for 15 minutes. Serve on a bed of Thai Rice and garnish with sesame seeds.

NUTRITIONAL INFORMATION PER PORTION			
Fat (g)	Carbohydrate (g)	Protein (g)	Energy (Cal)
13	8	57	392

Quick & Convenient Alternatives
Royco Mild Thai Curry Flavour Fiesta Sauce – packet

Chicken & Mushroom Supreme

SERVES 6

Heart Smart ◆ Diabetic

6–8 chicken breasts, skin and excess fat removed
1 clove garlic, crushed
15 ml (1 tbsp) chicken spice
5 ml (1 tsp) dried oreganum or
15 ml (1 tbsp) freshly chopped oreganum
1 onion, sliced
half a green pepper, cut into rings
1 x 397-g can mushroom soup
5 ml (1 tsp) curry powder

Rub the chicken pieces with garlic to coat and sprinkle with chicken spice and oreganum. Place the chicken pieces into a casserole dish and top with onion slices and green pepper rings. Mix the mushroom soup and curry powder together and pour over chicken. Bake, covered, at 180 °C for 45–60 minutes until cooked and tender. Serve a bed of wild or brown rice.

NUTRITIONAL INFORMATION PER PORTION			
Fat (g)	Carbohydrate (g)	Protein (g)	Energy (Cal)
7	3	26	190

Quick & Convenient Alternatives

Woolworths Mushroom & White Wine Cook-in-Sauce – can
Denny Garlic Mushroom Sauce – can
Walnut Ridge Mmm ... Fresh Mushroom Sauce – ready-made

Honey Mustard Chicken

SERVES 4

Heart Smart ◆ Diabetic

5 ml (1 tsp) curry powder
1 cube chicken stock
250 ml (1 cup) boiling water
30 ml (2 tbsp) mustard powder
60 ml (¼ cup) (4 tbsp) honey
30 ml (2 tbsp) lemon juice
6 chicken breasts, skin and excess fat removed
125 ml (½ cup) fat-free plain yoghurt
5–10 ml (1–2 tsp) cornflour
orange slices

Mix together the curry powder, stock cube, water, mustard, honey and lemon juice and cook over low heat for 5–10 minutes. Place the chicken pieces in a casserole dish and cover with the sauce. Bake, covered, at 180 °C, for 1–1½ hours until the chicken is cooked. Pour the sauce off, while straining, and set aside, returning the chicken, uncovered, to the oven for a further 15 minutes. Meanwhile, stir the yoghurt into the chicken sauce. Adjust the consistency of the sauce by adding more water if it is too thick, or thicken it with cornflour. Cover the chicken with the sauce and garnish with orange slices. Serve on bed of wild or brown rice.

NUTRITIONAL INFORMATION PER PORTION			
Fat (g)	Carbohydrate (g)	Protein (g)	Energy (Cal)
13	32	49	446

Citrus Chicken with Cointreau

SERVES 4

Heart Smart ◆ Diabetic

4–6 chicken breasts, skin removed, cut into cubes
125 ml (½ cup) thick cut marmalade
125 ml (½ cup) orange juice
250 ml (1 cup) French salad dressing
1 packet brown onion soup
1 orange, sliced
25 ml (1 tot) Cointreau

Mix all the ingredients together, except the orange slices and Cointreau. Place in a casserole dish and cook, covered, at 180 °C for 25–30 minutes or until cooked. Pour the Cointreau over just before serving and garnish with orange slices. Serve with wild rice and crisp tossed salad.

NUTRITIONAL INFORMATION PER PORTION			
Fat (g)	Carbohydrate (g)	Protein (g)	Energy (Cal)
16	39	31	437

Mediterranean Chicken

SERVES 4

Heart Smart ◆ Diabetic◆ Microwave

4–6 chicken breasts, skin removed
250 ml (1 cup) stock
2 large leeks, thinly sliced
2 cloves garlic
1 green pepper, seeded and diced
2 courgettes, trimmed and sliced
1 large aubergine, diced and rinsed once cut
4 large ripe tomatoes, chopped
25 ml (1 heaped tbsp) tomato paste
15 ml (1 tbsp) sugar
salt and freshly ground black pepper
15 ml (1 tbsp) freshly chopped oreganum or basil

Place the chicken pieces and 2 tbsp of the stock into a microwave dish and cover. Cook on medium power (75%) for 6–8 minutes, then set aside. Brown the leeks and the garlic in a little of the stock. Add the chicken and the remaining ingredients and simmer, covered, for 45 minutes. Season and add herbs. If the mixture is too dry, add more stock; if it is too watery, thicken it with 1–2 tsp cornflour mixed to a thin paste in a little water. Serve with noodles.

NUTRITIONAL INFORMATION PER PORTION			
Fat	**Carbohydrate**	**Protein**	**Energy**
(g)	(g)	(g)	(Cal)
10	13	41	323

Quick & Convenient Alternatives
Pick 'n Pay Choice Tomato & Onion Mix
Woolworths Mediterranean Tomato Cook-in-Sauce – can
Woolworths Char-Grilled Vegetables in Tomato Sauce – fresh

Yoghurt Chicken Casserole
SERVES 4

Heart Smart ◆ Diabetic

4–6 chicken pieces, skin removed
1 onion, chopped
1 clove garlic, crushed
2 ml (½ tsp) cayenne pepper
salt and ground pepper to taste
125 ml (½ cup) chicken stock
200 ml (¾ cup) fat-free plain yoghurt or buttermilk
45 ml (3 tbsp) skimmed milk
5 ml (1 tsp) paprika

Cook the chicken, onion, garlic, cayenne pepper, salt and pepper in a little stock, sherry or wine until browned. Add the stock and simmer for about 20 minutes, until the chicken is tender. Remove from the heat and stir in the milk and yoghurt. Heat through. Sprinkle with paprika and serve with a baked potato and seasonal vegetables.

NUTRITIONAL INFORMATION PER PORTION			
Fat (g)	Carbohydrate (g)	Protein (g)	Energy (Cal)
7	4	30	204

DIETICIAN'S TIP
Cultured buttermilk is made from skim milk with the addition of bacterial cultures giving it a more acidic, sharper flavour than Bulgarian yoghurt. Its fat content is generally less than 2%.

Chinese 3-Cup Chicken
SERVES 4

Heart Smart ◆ Diabetic

4–6 chicken breast fillets, skin removed
250 ml (1 cup) water
250 ml (1 cup) sherry
250 ml (1 cup) soy sauce
2 cloves garlic, peeled and crushed
2 cm fresh root ginger,
peeled and finely grated
30 ml (2 tbsp) sugar

Keeping the chicken breasts aside, combine all the ingredients to make up the sauce. Now cook the chicken in half the sauce until just done, then remove the chicken and set aside. Add the remaining sauce and simmer until the sauce develops a sticky consistency. Add the chicken to the sauce again, and allow to heat through. Serve immediately on a bed of wild rice or noodles.

NUTRITIONAL INFORMATION PER PORTION			
Fat	Carbohydrate	Protein	Energy
(g)	(g)	(g)	(Cal)
7	16	33	313

Quick & Convenient Alternatives
Walnut Ridge Chinese Sweet 'n Sour Dining In Sauce – ready-made
Ina Paarman Apple & Soy Sauce – ready-made
Woolworths Sweet & Spicy Grill & Bake Sauce – ready-made
All Gold Sweet 'n Sour Cook-in-Sauce – can
Woolworths Sweet 'n Sour Sauce – fresh

FISH & SEAFOOD

Thai Fish Bites
SERVES 4

Heart Smart ◆ Diabetic

10 ml (2 tsp) turmeric
5 ml (1 tsp) dried tarragon or marjoram, or
15 ml (1 tbsp) freshly chopped tarragon or marjoram
5 ml (1 tsp) salt
750 g hake or kingklip fillets,
skinned and cut into bite-sized pieces
1 large onion, chopped
1 clove garlic, crushed
1 chilli, finely chopped
4 cm fresh root ginger, peeled and chopped
5 ml (1 tsp) freshly chopped lemon grass
or finely grated lemon rind
5 ml (1 tsp) sugar
1 x 410-g can tomatoes or 3 large tomatoes, chopped
1 x 440-g can pineapple pieces

Mix the turmeric, herbs and salt and rub onto fish fillets. Heat a non-stick frying pan or one prepared with Spray and Cook, and cook the fish pieces for 2 minutes on each side. Remove the fish and set aside. Cook the onion, garlic, chilli, ginger and lemon grass in the pan with a little water or sherry to prevent sticking. Stir in the sugar, tomatoes and pineapple pieces. Cover and simmer for 10 minutes. Add the fish and allow to heat through – do not stir. Serve immediately on a bed of noodles.

NUTRITIONAL INFORMATION PER PORTION			
Fat (g)	Carbohydrate (g)	Protein (g)	Energy (Cal)
2	12	49	273

Quick & Convenienct Alternative

Woolworths Sweet 'n Spicy Grill & Bake Sauce – ready-made
Woolworths Sweet 'n Sour Pineapple and Lemon Sauce for
Vegetables – ready-made
Royco Sweet 'n Sour Sauce – packet
All Gold Sweet 'n Sour Cook-in-Sauce – can
Walnut Ridge Chinese Sweet 'n Sour Dining In Sauce – ready-made

Herbed Salmon Fillets

SERVES 4

Heart Smart ◆ Diabetic

700 g salmon fillets, skinned and cut into
4 evenly sized pieces
5 ml (1 tsp) dried mixed herbs,
or 15 ml (1 tbsp) freshly chopped mixed herbs
1 clove garlic, crushed
45 ml (3 tbsp) dry white wine
45 ml (3 tbsp) chicken stock
half a small red pepper, sliced
6–8 black olives, pitted and halved
ground black pepper to taste

Place the salmon, herbs and garlic in a shallow pan. Pour the wine and
stock over the fish and cook over medium heat for 2–3 minutes. Reduce
the heat and add the remaining ingredients. Cover and cook for a further
5–8 minutes. Serve on a bed of mashed potato with seasonal vegetables.

NUTRITIONAL INFORMATION PER PORTION			
Fat (g)	Carbohydrate (g)	Protein (g)	Energy (Cal)
14	1	36	290

Mixed Seafood Stir-Fry

SERVES 6

Heart Smart ◆ Diabetic

625 g kabeljou/red roman fillets, cubed
1 large onion, sliced
2 sticks celery, chopped
125 ml (½ cup) chicken stock
100 g shellfish of your choice
65 g (½ punnet) mixed sprouts
15 ml (1 tbsp) sherry
15 ml (1 tbsp) soy sauce
15 ml (1 tbsp) lemon juice
vegetables as desired

Lightly cook the fish cubes, onion and celery in a little stock, and set aside. Cook the remaining ingredients, including the shellfish, in a wok or large deep pot, tossing continuously, until tender. Add the fish mixture a few minutes before the end of cooking time to allow the fish to heat through. Serve with wild or brown rice.

NUTRITIONAL INFORMATION PER PORTION			
Fat (g)	Carbohydrate (g)	Protein (g)	Energy (Cal)
1	6	32	177

Quick & Convenient Alternatives
Pick 'n Pay Seafood Mix – frozen
Woolworths Vegetables with Sweet 'n Sour Sauce Stir-Fry
Woolworths Stir-Fry Range – fresh
Pick 'n Pay Hake in Sweet 'n Sour Sauce – frozen
Pick 'n Pay Choice Stir-Fry Range – frozen
Pick 'n Pay Foodhall Stir-Fry Range – fresh
Table Top Stir-Fry Range – frozen

Stuffed Calamari Casserole
SERVES 4

Heart Smart ◆ Diabetic

8 slices stale whole-wheat bread,
crusts removed and crumbed
1 clove garlic, peeled and crushed
5 ml (1 tsp) dried parsley
3 ml (½ tsp) garlic and herb seasoning
1 egg, beaten (optional)
1 x 410-g can tomato mix
300 g calamari tubes

Combine the ingredients to make up the stuffing, and stuff the calamari tubes. Arrange these in a casserole dish and pour the tomato mix over. Cover and bake at 160 °C for 30–40 minutes.

NUTRITIONAL INFORMATION PER PORTION			
Fat (g)	Carbohydrate (g)	Protein (g)	Energy (Cal)
3	48	22	305

Quick & Convenient Alternative
All Gold Chopped Tomato Mix – can
All Gold Natural Fresh Cut Diced Peeled Tomato – can
Pick 'n Pay Choice Italian Classic Chopped Peeled Tomato – can

---

CHEF'S TIP

The golden rule when cooking calamari rings is either to use quick, dry, hot frying as a cooking method or, as used in this case, long, slow, moist cooking to ensure a tender cooked product.

Seafood Paella

SERVES 4–6

Heart Smart ◆ Diabetic

250 ml (1 cup) uncooked brown rice
1 onion, peeled and chopped
3 rashers lean back bacon,
fat trimmed and finely chopped
125 ml (½ cup) dry white wine
125 ml (½ cup) stock
1 clove garlic, peeled and crushed
30 ml (2 tbsp) lemon juice
5 ml (1 tsp) freshly chopped marjoram
5 ml (1 tsp) freshly chopped oreganum
150 g calamari
150 g shrimps or small prawns
250 ml (1 cup) mushrooms, cleaned and sliced
125 ml (½ cup) frozen peas
vegetables of your choice, chopped
or broken into bite-sized pieces
salt and pepper to taste

Cook the rice according to the manufacturer's instructions, and set aside. Cook the onion and bacon in a little wine or stock for a few minutes. Now add the remaining wine and stock, the garlic, lemon juice, herbs, calamari and shrimps/prawns. Simmer, uncovered, until almost all the liquid has evaporated. Add the mushrooms, peas and other vegetables. Cook until the vegetables are tender, adding more liquid as necessary. Add the rice and allow to heat through. Garnish with fresh tomato slices and parsley.

NUTRITIONAL INFORMATION PER PORTION			
Fat (g)	Carbohydrate (g)	Protein (g)	Energy (Cal)
2	26	18	297

Fisherman's Pie
SERVES 4

Heart Smart ◆ Diabetic

500 g fresh tuna or haddock, skinned and deboned
250 ml (1 cup) skimmed milk
1 bay leaf
15 ml (1 tbsp) cornflour
5 ml (1 tsp) stock powder
15 ml (1 tbsp) freshly chopped herbs of your choice
120 g (1 cup) cooked peas
250 g (1 cup) mushrooms, sliced
4 large potatoes, cooked and mashed
60 g (3 tbsp) fat-free cottage cheese
some skimmed milk if the mixture is too stiff
salt and pepper to taste

Poach the fish in a cup of milk, together with the bay leaf, until tender. Remove the fish, flake and set aside. Remove the bay leaf and discard, reserving the milk. Mix the cornflour and stock powder to a paste with a little water or milk. Bring the milk used for the poaching to the boil and add the cornflour paste. Stir until thickened. Add the herbs, peas and mushrooms. Layer the cooked fish in a casserole dish, cover with sauce and set aside. Mash together the potatoes, cottage cheese and extra skimmed milk if necessary. Season this mixture to taste and spread over the fish. Bake at 180 °C for 20 minutes. Garnish with a twist of lemon and serve with a tossed green salad.

NUTRITIONAL INFORMATION PER PORTION			
Fat (g)	Carbohydrate (g)	Protein (g)	Energy (Cal)
2	32	40	323

Quick & Convenient Alternative
Country Herb Smash – packet

Spanish Tuna Casserole

SERVES 4

Heart Smart ◆ Diabetic

1 large onion, peeled and chopped
4 cloves garlic, peeled and crushed
1 large red pepper, seeded and cut into julienne strips
1 large green pepper, seeded and cut into julienne strips
250 ml (1 cup) dry white wine
1 fresh chilli, seeded and cut into julienne strips
salt and freshly ground black pepper
10 ml (2 tsp) paprika
1 x 410 g-can whole peeled tomatoes, drained and chopped
3 medium potatoes, peeled and diced into 1.5-cm cubes
600 g fresh tuna, cleaned and cut into 3-cm chunks
juice of 1 lemon
5 ml (1 tsp) freshly chopped dill or thyme

Cook the onion, garlic and peppers in a little wine until soft. Add the chilli, salt, pepper, paprika and tomatoes and allow to simmer for 10 minutes. Add the potatoes and the rest of the wine and cook, covered, for 25–30 minutes. Meanwhile, drizzle the fish chunks with lemon juice and season with salt, pepper and herbs. Check that the potatoes are cooked, then add the fish to the casserole. Cover and cook for a further 5 minutes. Serve with hot, crusty white bread.

NUTRITIONAL INFORMATION PER PORTION			
Fat (g)	Carbohydrate (g)	Protein (g)	Energy (Cal)
2	27	42	348

Hasty Hake Bake
SERVES 6

Heart Smart ◆ Diabetic

500 g fresh hake fillets, skinned
400 g (2 cups) fresh/frozen mixed vegetables
1 packet white onion or mushroom soup (powder)
250 ml (1 cup) skimmed milk

Arrange the hake fillets in an ovenproof dish. Spread the mixed vegetables evenly on top. Mix the soup powder and milk together and pour this over the vegetables. Bake at 180 °C for about an hour.

NUTRITIONAL INFORMATION PER PORTION			
Fat	**Carbohydrate**	**Protein**	**Energy**
(g)	(g)	(g)	(Cal)
1	9	25	155

CHEF'S TIP
Chillies and peppers both belong to the Capsicum family. Their flavour generally becomes sweeter as the colour changes from green to red, orange and yellow. When trying to determine how hot the chilli will be, the size rather than the colour is the important factor. It is believed that the smaller the chilli, the hotter it will be.

MEAT

Ostrich Chilli Con Carne
SERVES 2–4

Heart Smart ◆ Diabetic

1 small onion, chopped
half a green pepper, seeded and chopped
1 clove garlic, crushed
250 ml (1 cup) stock
200 g ostrich mince
2–3 leaves fresh basil, finely chopped
1 bay leaf
freshly chopped chilli to taste
salt and pepper to taste
1 x 410-g can tomatoes
200 g (1 cup) kidney beans, cooked

Cook the onion, green pepper and garlic in a little stock until tender. Add the mince, herbs and seasoning and allow the mince to brown. Add the remaining stock and the tomatoes, and bring to the boil. Then reduce the heat and simmer, uncovered, until the sauce has thickened and reduced in quantity by half. Add the kidney beans and heat through. Serve on a bed of wild or brown rice.

NUTRITIONAL INFORMATION PER PORTION			
Fat (g)	Carbohydrate (g)	Protein (g)	Energy (Cal)
3	17	21	198

Quick & Convenient Alternatives
Walnut Ridge Tomato & Basil Sauce – ready-made
Pick 'n Pay Choice Chopped Peeled Tomato with Chilli – can

Walnut Lamb

SERVES 4

Heart Smart ◆ Diabetic

450 g boned leg of lamb, fat trimmed and cubed
2 onions, sliced
1 clove garlic, crushed
250 ml (1 cup) pineapple juice
45 ml (3 tbsp) tomato paste
30 ml (2 tbsp) vinegar
10 ml (2 tsp) soy sauce
15 ml (1 tbsp) sugar
2 ml (½ tsp) curry powder
4 thin strips lemon peel
60 ml (¼ cup) walnuts
freshly ground black pepper

Brown the meat, onion and garlic in a saucepan with a little pineapple juice. Add all the other ingredients – except the walnuts – and simmer for 5–10 minutes. Place in a casserole dish, sprinkle with walnuts and cook at 180 °C for an hour. Serve on a bed of raisin rice.

NUTRITIONAL INFORMATION PER PORTION			
Fat (g)	Carbohydrate (g)	Protein (g)	Energy (Cal)
15	19	35	350

Beef & Prune Casserole

SERVES 6–8

Heart Smart ◆ Diabetic

3 onions, chopped
3 cloves garlic, crushed
2 sticks celery, chopped
1 kg beef shin, cubed, fat trimmed
1.5 litres beef stock
15 ml (3 tsp) coriander, ground
5 ml (1 tsp) allspice
5 ml (1 tsp) chilli powder
30 ml (2 tbsp) wine vinegar
250 g prunes, soaked and stoned
2 bay leaves
2 mealies, stripped from the cob
salt and pepper to taste
200 ml (¾ cup) fat-free plain yoghurt
5 ml (1 tsp) chopped parsley

Cook onions, garlic, celery and meat until browned and tender, in a little of the stock. Add the spices, chilli powder and vinegar and cook for a further 2–3 minutes. Add the prunes, bay leaves, mealies and remaining stock and bring to the boil. Reduce heat and simmer, covered, for 1½ hours. Stir occasionally and season to taste. Stir in the yoghurt just before serving and garnish with parsley.

NUTRITIONAL INFORMATION PER PORTION			
Fat	Carbohydrate	Protein	Energy
(g)	(g)	(g)	(Cal)
14	32	49	458

Quick & Convenient Alternative
Walnut Ridge Brewers Beef Incredible Casserole – ready-made

Spiced Minced Beef with Spinach Rice

SERVES 4–6

Heart Smart ◆ Diabetic

700 g extra lean minced beef
500–625 ml (2–2½ cups) beef stock
1 large onion, peeled and chopped
2 cloves garlic, peeled and crushed
5 ml (1 tsp) ground turmeric
5 ml (1 tsp) ground cumin
5 ml (1 tsp) ground coriander
5 ml (1 tsp) garam masala
175 g spinach, roughly chopped
350 g (2⅔ cups) cooked basmati rice
(this is about 200 g or 1 cup uncooked basmati rice)
125 ml (½ cup) sultanas
60 ml (¼ cup) almonds (optional)

Brown the mince in a little stock, sherry or wine over low heat, then add the onion, garlic and spices. Cook for 6–8 minutes. Add the remaining stock and bring to the boil, then cover and simmer for 20 minutes. Add the spinach and cooked rice to the meat mixture, allowing the spinach leaves to wilt and the rice to heat through. Stir in the sultanas and almonds. Serve with fresh vegetables.

NUTRITIONAL INFORMATION PER PORTION			
Fat	**Carbohydrate**	**Protein**	**Energy**
(g)	(g)	(g)	(Cal)
12	31	42	333

Quick & Convenient Alternative
Tastic Wild Spinach & Onion Savoury Classic – box

Spicy South African Bobotie

SERVES 4–6

Heart Smart ◆ Diabetic

1 onion, peeled and chopped
1 clove garlic, peeled and crushed
1 apple, peeled, cored and diced
35 ml (2½ tbsp) skim milk
1 thick slice of bread
500 g extra lean beef mince or ostrich mince
15 ml (1 tbsp) curry powder
30 ml (2 tbsp) sugar
15 ml (1 tbsp) apricot jam
5 ml (1 tsp) salt
25 ml (2 tbsp) raisins
60 ml (4 tbsp) vinegar
2 bay leaves
5 ml (1 tsp) turmeric
2 eggs, beaten with 2 tbsp skim milk
and a pinch of nutmeg

Brown the onion, garlic and apple in a little stock, sherry or wine over low heat. Meanwhile, soak the bread in the milk. Mix the remaining ingredients together, with the exception of the eggs, milk and nutmeg, and add the onion mixture, as well as the soaked bread. Cook for 8–10 minutes over moderate heat. Beat the eggs, milk and nutmeg together and set aside. Line an ovenproof dish with the meat mixture, then cover with the beaten egg mixture. Cook at 180 ˚C until the egg is set and golden brown. Serve with fresh vegetables and yellow rice.

NUTRITIONAL INFORMATION PER PORTION			
Fat (g)	Carbohydrate (g)	Protein (g)	Energy (Cal)
6	22	25	238

Chinese Sweet 'n Sour Pork

SERVES 4

Heart Smart ◆ Diabetic

450 g boneless pork loin chops, fat trimmed,
cut into 15 mm-wide strips
1 clove garlic, peeled and crushed
75 g button mushrooms, washed and left whole
1.5 cm fresh root ginger, peeled and finely grated
125 ml (½ cup) chicken stock
85 ml (⅓ cup) dry sherry
1 small red pepper, cut into strips
1 small green pepper, cut into strips
30 ml (2 tbsp) soy sauce
1 x 440-g can pineapple pieces, crained
2 ml (¼ tsp) cinnamon
2 ml (¼ tsp) ground coriander
45 ml (3 tbsp) fat-free plain yoghurt or buttermilk
30 ml (2 tbsp) fruit chutney
15 ml (1 tbsp) cornflour

Cook the pork strips, garlic, mushrooms and ginger in a little stock for 10 minutes. Add the sherry, remaining stock, peppers, soy sauce, pineapple pieces and spices. Cook for a further 5–8 minutes, then stir in the yoghurt/buttermilk and chutney. If necessary, thicken with cornflour by mixing to a paste with a little fluid before adding to the dish.

NUTRITIONAL INFORMATION PER PORTION			
Fat (g)	Carbohydrate (g)	Protein (g)	Energy (Cal)
13	30	34	395

Quick & Convenient Alternatives
Royco Sweet 'n Sour Sauce – packet
Woolworths Oriental Sweet 'n Sour Cook-in-Sauce – can
Amoy Sweet 'n Sour Sauce – bottle

Mexican Steak

SERVES 4

Heart Smart ◆ Diabetic

**4 ostrich steaks, 20–25 mm thick
10 ml (2 tsp) salt
65 ml (¼ cup) orange juice
65 ml (¼ cup) tomato juice
30 ml (2 tbsp) lemon juice
30 ml (40 g) (2 tbsp) fruit chutney
30 ml (2 tbsp) peri-peri sauce of your choice
5 ml (1 tsp) paprika
1–2 cloves garlic, crushed**

Mix all the ingredients to make up a marinade, and marinate the meat, covered, for 4–6 hours in the refrigerator. Place the steaks on a grid over coals or in a pre-heated oven, and grill to the required degree – for a medium rare steak, count on this taking about 10–15 minutes. Serve with baked potatoes and seasonal vegetables.

NUTRITIONAL INFORMATION PER PORTION			
Fat	**Carbohydrate**	**Protein**	**Energy**
(g)	(g)	(g)	(Cal)
4	8	26	167

Quick & Convenient Alternatives
Steers Peri-Peri Sauce – bottle
Wellington Chilli Sauces – bottle
Crosse & Blackwell Chilli Sauce – bottle

Fruity Ostrich Casserole

SERVES 4

Heart Smart ♦ Diabetic

500 g ostrich meat for stewing
2 onions, chopped
375 ml (1½ cups) beef stock
5 ml (1 tsp) salt
a pinch of ground black pepper
5 ml (1 tsp) dried oreganum or
15 ml (3 tsp) fresh oreganum
125 g dried apricots, chopped
125 g prunes, pitted and chopped
15 ml (1 tbsp) soy sauce
30 ml (2 tbsp) wine vinegar

Cook the meat and onion in a little stock over medium heat until brown. Add all the remaining ingredients. Simmer for about an hour or until the meat is tender. Serve on a bed of rice with crisp seasonal vegetables.

NUTRITIONAL INFORMATION PER PORTION			
Fat	Carbohydrate	Protein	Energy
(g)	(g)	(g)	(Cal)
4	36	29	297

Quick & Convenient Alternative
Walnut Ridge Savoury Farmstyle Apricot Unbelievable
Chicken – ready-made

Pork Curry

SERVES 4

Heart Smart ◆ Diabetic

450 g lean pork fillet, fat trimmed and diced
1 clove garlic, crushed
1 onion, sliced
2 sticks celery, sliced
2 large carrots, cleaned and sliced
500 ml (2 cups) beef stock
15 ml (1 tbsp) curry powder
5 ml (1 tsp) ground cumin
5 ml (1 tsp) ground coriander
2 ml (½ tsp) garam masala
2 ml (½ tsp) ground cardamom
2 ml (½ tsp) turmeric
175 g green beans, trimmed and halved
100 g (1 cup) raisins
2 courgettes, sliced
175 ml (1 small tub) low-fat plain yoghurt

Cook the pork, garlic, onion, celery and carrots in a little stock for 5–10 minutes. Add the spices and remaining stock and simmer, covered, for 45 minutes to an hour until tender. Add beans, raisins and courgettes and cook for another 10 minutes until tender. Remove from heat and stir in the yoghurt. Serve with rice and fruit chutney.

NUTRITIONAL INFORMATION PER PORTION			
Fat (g)	Carbohydrate (g)	Protein (g)	Energy (Cal)
13	30	38	400

Quick & Convenient Alternatives
All Gold Spicy Curry Cook-in-Sauce – can
Royco Chutney Curry Sauce Sensation – packet
Woolworths Durban Curry Cook-in-Sauce – can
Walnut Ridge Mild Fruity Irresistible Curry – ready-made
Ina Paarman Spicy Curry Sauce – ready-made

Lebanese Koosa
SERVES 6

Heart Smart ◆ Diabetic

12 large courgettes (each with a diameter of 4–5 cm)
125 g ostrich mince
125 ml (½ cup) uncooked rice
5 ml (1 tsp) nutmeg
salt and pepper to taste
2 x 410-g cans chopped tomatoes
half a cup of boiling water

Rinse the courgettes, and use a sharp knife to remove only the ends where the stalks were attached. Now hollow out the courgettes using an apple corer – leaving the closed ends of the courgettes intact – and place the flesh that has been removed into the bottom of a deep casserole dish. Mix together the mince, rice, nutmeg and seasoning. Stuff the hollowed out courgettes with the mince mixture and layer this on top of the courgette flesh. Scatter the remaining mince mixture on top and pour the tomatoes over this, together with half a cup of boiling water. Bake at 180 °C for an hour.

NUTRITIONAL INFORMATION PER PORTION			
Fat	Carbohydrate	Protein	Energy
(g)	(g)	(g)	(Cal)
2	22	9	148

Veal Stir-Fry

SERVES 6

Heart Smart ◆ Diabetic

1 clove garlic, peeled and finedly chopped
5 ml (1 tsp) fresh root ginger,
peeled and finely chopped
500 g veal fillet, cut into strips
15 ml (1 tbsp) soy sauce
15 ml (1 tbsp) sherry/brandy
5 ml (1 tsp) salt
5 ml (1 tsp) sugar
5 ml (1 tsp) cornflour
5 ml (1 tsp) vegetable oil
2 carrots, cut into strips
half a bunch of spring onions, chopped
half a red pepper, seeded and cut into strips
half a green pepper, seeded and cut into strips
half a small cabbage, shredded
1 stalk celery, sliced
250 g mushrooms, sliced
2 slices fresh pineapple, coarsely chopped
100 g mixed sprouts
125 ml (½ cup) stock
pepper to taste

Mix the garlic, ginger, meat, soy sauce, sherry/brandy, salt, sugar and cornflour, and cook in the oil for 15–20 minutes. Add the remaining ingredients and half the stock, and cook until tender and heated through. Add more stock as required. Season to taste, and serve on a bed of rice.

NUTRITIONAL INFORMATION PER PORTION			
Fat (g)	Carbohydrate (g)	Protein (g)	Energy (Cal)
7	9	30	231

Quick Cottage Pie

SERVES 4–6

Heart Smart ◆ Diabetic

450 g extra lean beef mince/ostrich mince
125 ml (½ cup) stock
1 large onion, peeled and chopped
1 large carrot, peeled and grated
1 x 410-g can tomatoes
or three ripe tomatoes, chopped
30 ml (2 tbsp) tomato paste
5 ml (1 tsp) allspice
5 ml (1 tsp) mixed herbs
15 ml (1 tbsp) Worcestershire sauce
4 large potatoes
5 ml (1 tsp) mustard powder
salt and pepper to taste
5 ml (1 tsp) baking powder
60 ml (¼ cup) skimmed milk
15 ml (1 tbsp) sesame seeds (optional)

Cook the mince in a little stock over low heat until browned, then add the onion and carrot and cook for a further 5–6 minutes. Stir in the tomatoes, tomato paste, allspice, remaining stock, herbs and Worcestershire sauce, and cook for a further 20 minutes. Meanwhile, cook the potatoes in boiling, salted water or in the microwave until soft. Mash, and add the mustard powder, salt, pepper, baking powder and milk. Spoon the meat mixture into an ovenproof dish and place a layer of the mashed potato mixture on top. Fluff with a fork, sprinkle with sesame seeds and brown under the grill until golden.

NUTRITIONAL INFORMATION PER PORTION			
Fat (g)	Carbohydrate (g)	Protein (g)	Energy (Cal)
8	25	28	255

VEGETARIAN DISHES

Spicy Vegetable & Chickpea Curry
SERVES 4

Vegetarian ◆ Heart Smart ◆ Diabetic

15 ml (1 tbsp) vegetable oil
5 ml (1 tsp) cumin seeds
2 sticks cinnamon
2 cloves
1 large onion, peeled and chopped
1 clove garlic, crushed
3 cm fresh root ginger, peeled and finely grated
2 red chillies, finely chopped or minced
15 ml (1 tbsp) freshly chopped coriander leaves
10 ml (2 tsp) turmeric
5 ml (1 tsp) salt
4 medium potatoes (about 450 g), cut into cubes
250 ml (1 cup) frozen peas
1 x 397-g can chickpeas or red kidney beans, drained
1 small cauliflower, broken into florets
1 x 410-g can tomatoes
5–10 ml (1–2 tsp) cornflour

Heat the oil and add the cumin seeds, cinnamon and cloves. Allow to sizzle for a minute. Add the onion, garlic, ginger, chillies, coriander, turmeric and salt, stirring gently until the onion is translucent. Add all the vegetables and the tomatoes, cover and cook gently over moderate heat until tender. Adjust the consistency by adding cornflour to thicken the mixture if necessary. Garnish with freshly chopped coriander leaves and serve on a bed of rice with poppadums.

NUTRITIONAL INFORMATION PER PORTION			
Fat (g)	Carbohydrate (g)	Protein (g)	Energy (Cal)
5	47	15	329

Quick & Convenient Alternatives
All Gold Spicy Curry Cook-in-Sauce – can
Walnut Ridge Mild Fruity Irresistable Curry – ready-made
Woolworths Cape Malay Curry Cook-in-Sauce – can

Lentil Stew
SERVES 4–6

Vegetarian ◆ Heart Smart ◆ Diabetic

2 small onions, peeled and chopped
2 cloves garlic, peeled and crushed
1 small red pepper, seeded and chopped
4 courgettes, sliced
1 large carrot, grated
1 large aubergine, diced
250 ml (1 cup) tomato purée
15 ml (1 tbsp) honey
30 ml (2 tbsp) soy sauce
60 ml (¼ cup) freshly chopped parsley
15 ml (1 tbsp) freshly chopped basil
250 ml (1 cup) water
1 litre (4 cups) cooked lentils
salt and pepper to taste

Cook the onion, garlic, pepper, courgettes and carrot in a little stock over low heat for 5 minutes. Add the remaining ingredients, except the lentils, cover and simmer for 30 minutes. Add the cooked lentils and more water as required. Simmer for another 15 minutes and season to taste. Serve with brown rice and top with a sprinkling of grated cheese.

NUTRITIONAL INFORMATION PER PORTION			
Fat	Carbohydrate	Protein	Energy
(g)	(g)	(g)	(Cal)
1	50	16	255

Quick & Convenient Alternative
Pick 'n Pay Choice Italian Classic Original Passata Sauce – bottled

Rich Bean & Vegetable Casserole
SERVES 4–6

Vegetarian ◆ Heart Smart ◆ Diabetic

1 onion, peeled and chopped
2 cloves garlic, crushed
2 sticks celery, sliced
1 x 410-g can chopped tomatoes
45 ml (3 tbsp) tomato paste
5 ml (1 tsp) honey or sugar
500 ml (2 cups) vegetable stock
3 ml (½ tsp) coriander
3 ml (½ tsp) allspice
3 ml (½ tsp) cayenne pepper
2 bay leaves
2 aubergines, cubed
100 g mangetout, trimmed and halved
100 g baby corn, halved
3 courgettes, sliced
2 medium carrots, sliced
salt and pepper to taste
5 ml (1 tsp) dried basil, or
5 ml (1 tbsp) freshly chopped basil
225 g cannellini beans, cooked
225 g red kidney beans, cooked

Place all the ingredients, with the exception of the basil and the beans, in a deep saucepan and simmer for 30 minutes or until the vegetables are tender, but still firm. Add seasoning to taste, and add the beans and the basil. Cook for a further 8–10 minutes and serve on a bed of rice.

NUTRITIONAL INFORMATION PER PORTION			
Fat (g)	Carbohydrate (g)	Protein (g)	Energy (Cal)
2	35	12	240

CHEF'S TIP
This recipe is equally successful when you use only half the amount of beans.

Basil & Tomato Risotto
SERVES 4

Vegetarian ◆ Heart Smart ◆ Diabetic

75 g broccoli, cut into very small florets
1 onion, peeled and chopped
4 large ripe tomatoes, chopped
30 ml (2 tbsp) lemon juice
500 ml (2 cups) button mushrooms, halved
5 ml (1 tsp) dried basil,
or 15 ml (1 tbsp) freshly chopped basil
125 ml (½ cup) dry white wine
1 litre (4 cups) vegetable stock
125 ml (½ cup) risotto or arborio rice
125 ml (½ cup) brown lentils,
soaked in a cup of water overnight
Parmesan cheese

Lightly steam the broccoli over boiling water or in a microwave until tender, but firm. Set it aside. Mix the onion, tomatoes, lemon juice and mushrooms, and cook in a little stock until tender. Season, add the basil and the broccoli, then simmer for a further 3–5 minutes and set aside. Mix the wine and the stock, bring to the boil, and add the rice and the pre-soaked, drained lentils. Cover and simmer for 35 minutes, stirring occasionally until tender. Add the tomato mixture and stir to mix it into the rice. Sprinkle with Parmesan cheese and serve immediately with salad or vegetables.

NUTRITIONAL INFORMATION PER PORTION			
Fat (g)	Carbohydrate (g)	Protein (g)	Energy (Cal)
1	35	9	223

CHEF'S TIPS

For the pancakes on the following page, other suitable vegetarian fillings include: *peppadew and artichokes; peppers and courgette; mushrooms (will lose some water, so cook lightly first) and broccoli; onion, gherkin and tomato.*

Non-vegetarian fillings include: *lean back bacon with the visible fat removed; chopped lean sandwich ham; smoked snoek; tuna in brine.*

Greek Pancakes with Spinach & Feta

SERVES 4–6

Vegetarian ◆ Heart Smart ◆ Diabetic

FOR THE FILLING
250 g spinach, washed and shredded
the juice of 1 lemon
salt and freshly ground black pepper to taste
3 ml (½ tsp) nutmeg
30 ml (2 tbsp) olives, pitted and halved
5 marinated sun-dried tomatoes, chopped
175 ml (1 small tub) low-fat plain yoghurt
50 g feta cheese (8 blocks, each measuring 25 x 15 x 15 mm)

FOR THE PANCAKES
250 ml (1 cup) flour
1 egg, beaten
375 ml (1½ cups) skimmed milk

To make the filling: Steam the spinach leaves in lightly salted water until wilted. Drain and chop finely. Add all the remaining ingredients, mix thoroughly and allow to heat through.

To make the pancakes: Mix the ingredients together to form a smooth batter, then allow to stand for 20–30 minutes. Pour the batter into a hot, non-stick pan to a thickness of about 2 mm. Loosen the edges and flip onto the other side once bubbles appear on the surface and the dough cooks. Cook until golden brown. Fill the warm pancakes with the spinach filling, then roll up. Sprinkle with crumbled feta cheese and serve immediately

NUTRITIONAL INFORMATION PER PORTION			
Fat (g)	Carbohydrate (g)	Protein (g)	Energy (Cal)
5	32	12	222

Vegetarian Spaghetti Bolognaise
SERVES 4–6

Vegetarian ◆ Heart Smart ◆ Diabetic

250 ml (1 cup) unflavoured soya mince
750 ml (3 cups) boiling water
1 large onion, peeled and chopped
2 stalks celery, finely chopped
2 cloves garlic, peeled and crushed
60 ml (¼ cup) red wine
1 x 410-g can whole, peeled tomatoes
15 ml (1 tbsp) tomato paste
25 g (1 heaped tbsp) sugar
30 ml (2 tbsp) soy sauce
freshly chopped thyme, oreganum and basil
500 g (1 packet) spaghetti

Cover the soya mince with the water and leave to stand for 10 minutes.
Rinse the soya well in cold water. Cook the onion, celery and garlic in a
little of the wine until soft. Add all the other ingredients, including the
soya, but not the herbs. Cook gently for 20 minutes, adding the rest of the
wine or a little water. If necessary, thicken with a bit of cornflour or Bisto.
Add the herbs just before serving. Serve on a bed of spaghetti.

NUTRITIONAL INFORMATION PER PORTION			
Fat (g)	Carbohydrate (g)	Protein (g)	Energy (Cal)
9	80	25	499

Savoury Asparagus, Onion & Herb Tart

SERVES 4–6

Vegetarian ◆ Heart Smart ◆ Diabetic

215 g (or ½ x 430-g can) asparagus cuts, drained
1 onion, peeled and chopped
125 ml (½ cup) mature Cheddar cheese, grated
200 ml (⅔ cup) skimmed milk
30 ml (2 tbsp) flour
2 eggs, lightly beaten
5 ml (1 tsp) mustard powder
salt and pepper to taste
15 ml (1 tbsp) freshly chopped
marjoram or basil

As a filling, arrange the asparagus, onion and grated cheese in a pie dish sprayed with Spray and Cook. Combine all the remaining ingredients, with the exception of the herbs, and beat. Pour this over the filling in the pie dish and sprinkle with herbs. Bake at 180 °C for 30–40 minutes. Serve with fresh, crusty bread and crispy French salad.

NUTRITIONAL INFORMATION PER PORTION			
Fat	Carbohydrate	Protein	Energy
(g)	(g)	(g)	(Cal)
6	6	7	106

DIETICIAN'S TIP
Use an EXTRA mature Cheddar or blue cheese to add a stronger cheese flavour without adding too much extra fat.

Mexican Bean-Filled Tortillas

SERVES 6

Vegetarian ◆ Heart Smart ◆ Diabetic

FOR THE TORTILLAS
500 ml (2 cups) flour
5 ml (1 tsp) salt
1 egg, beaten
180 ml (¾ cup) cold water

FOR THE REFRIED BEANS
1 large tomato, chopped
1 small onion, peeled and chopped
1 clove garlic, peeled and crushed
1 x 410-g can red kidney beans, drained
1 fresh chilli, chopped
salt and pepper to taste

To make the tortillas: Sift together the dry ingredients. Beat the water and the egg together and stir enough of this mixture into the dry ingredients to form a soft dough. Knead the dough on a floured surface for about 10 minutes until it is smooth and elastic. Divide the dough into 12 pieces, rolling each into a 20-cm circle. Cook one at a time in a non-stick frying pan until brown spots appear on the underside and bubbles appear on the top surface. Turn over and cook on the other side, pressing the bubbles down with a spatula.

To make the refried beans: Cook the tomato, onion and garlic together. Stir in the beans and chilli and cook for 10 minutes. Season and fill the tortillas. Serve with salsa, guacamole and fresh salad

NUTRITIONAL INFORMATION PER PORTION			
Fat (g)	Carbohydrate (g)	Protein (g)	Energy (Cal)
2	53	10	297

DESSERTS

Baked Bananas
SERVES 4

Vegetarian ◆ Heart Smart ◆ Diabetic

4 bananas, peeled and sliced in half lenghthways
60 ml (4 tbsp) raisins
cinnamon
125 ml (½ cup) orange juice
125 ml (½ cup) rum

Place the bananas in a shallow, ovenproof dish and sprinkle with raisins and cinnamon. Add the fruit juice and the rum and bake at 180 °C for 30 minutes. Serve with fat-free, plain yoghurt and a drizzle of honey.

NUTRITIONAL INFORMATION PER PORTION			
Fat	Carbohydrate	Protein	Energy
(g)	(g)	(g)	(Cal)
1	33	1	215

Apple & Lemon Crumble
SERVES 4 – 6

Vegetarian ◆ Heart Smart ◆ Diabetic

6 apples (about 600 g) peeled, cored and sliced
1 lemon, juice and grated rind
125 ml (½ cup) wholemeal flour
125 ml (½ cup) oats
30 ml (2 tbsp) margarine
60 ml (¼ cup) soft brown sugar
60 ml (¼ cup) walnuts, chopped

Put the prepared apples into a deep, round ovenproof dish, add the lemon juice and mix. In a mixing bowl, mix together the flour and the oats and rub in the margarine. Stir in the sugar, nuts and lemon rind and spoon the mixture over the fruit. Bake at 180 °C for 25–30 minutes until the fruit is tender and the crumble is golden brown.

NUTRITIONAL INFORMATION PER PORTION			
Fat (g)	Carbohydrate (g)	Protein (g)	Energy (Cal)
7	44	5	263

Mango Dream
SERVES 4

Vegetarian ◆ Heart Smart ◆ Diabetic

15 ml (1 tbsp) custard powder
125 ml (½ cup) skimmed milk
30 ml (2 tbsp) sugar
175 ml (1 small tub) fat-free plain yoghurt
500 ml (2 cups) mango purée
or seasonal fruit purée
a sprig of mint to garnish

Make up the custard, using the milk and the sugar. Mix in the yoghurt and the fruit purée – blend until smooth. Chill and serve with fresh fruit slices. Garnish with a sprig of fresh mint.

NUTRITIONAL INFORMATION PER PORTION			
Fat (g)	Carbohydrate (g)	Protein (g)	Energy (Cal)
1	42	5	190

Pineapple Sorbet
SERVES 4

Vegetarian ◆ Heart Smart ◆ Diabetic

1 x 470-g tin crushed pineapple
5 ml (1 tsp) gelatine
1 small lemon, juice and finely grated rind
10 ml (2 tsp) sugar
175 ml (1 small tub) plain fat-free yoghurt
2 egg-whites, beaten until stiff
30 ml (2 tbsp) Cointreau (optional)

Drain the pineapple, keeping the juice, and set it aside. Melt the gelatine in a cup by mixing it with 2 tbsp hot water. Mix the pineapple juice with the lemon juice, sugar, gelatine and yoghurt. Freeze the mixture until ice crystals form throughout. Remove from the freezer and beat – ideally, using a food processor. Add the crushed pineapple, egg-whites and Cointreau (if using) and blend until smooth. Freeze for 24 hours or until frozen solid. Leave in the refrigerator for half an hour before serving. Serve garnished with fresh pineapple pieces and mint leaves.

NUTRITIONAL INFORMATION PER PORTION			
Fat	**Carbohydrate**	**Protein**	**Energy**
(g)	(g)	(g)	(Cal)
trace	30	5	150

Quick & Convenient Alternatives
Woolworths Slimmer's Choice Frozen Dessert
Weight-less Vanilla Dairy Dessert
Dun Robin Guilt-free Dairy Soft
Nestlé Dairymaid Country Fresh Lite
Aylesbury Classic Deluxe Sorbet Vanilla
Ola Diet Delight
Cas Diaby Ice Cream

Chocolate Cheesecake
SERVES 8–10

Vegetarian ♦ Heart Smart ♦ Diabetic

500 g (2 tubs) fat-free plain smooth cottage cheese
3 large eggs, lightly beaten
190 ml (¾ cup) sugar
5 ml (1 tsp) vanilla essence
10 ml (2 tsp) lemon juice
a pinch of salt
175 ml (1 small tub) plain fat-free yoghurt
50 g (1 small bar) plain dark chocolate
40 ml (3 tbsp) cocoa powder
3 ml (½ tsp) coffee powder
45 ml (3 tbsp) warm water

Blend together the cottage cheese, eggs, sugar, vanilla essence, lemon juice, yoghurt and salt. In a double-boiler melt the chocolate and mix in the cocoa, coffee and water. Beat until smooth and creamy. Pour the cheesecake mixture into the chocolate mixture and swirl to create a marbled effect. Pour into a greased or non-stick cake tin and bake at 180 °C for 40–45 minutes, ensuring that the cake tin rests in a pan of water during cooking. Allow the cake to cool for at least 12 hours before serving.

NUTRITIONAL INFORMATION PER PORTION			
Fat (g)	Carbohydrate (g)	Protein (g)	Energy (Cal)
4	24	11	176

CHEF'S TIP
To make the cheesecake less rich, a layered filling can be made using cream crackers or water biscuits.

Citrus Crème Caramel
SERVES 4

Vegetarian ◆ Heart Smart ◆ Diabetic

FOR THE CITRUS CARAMEL
125 ml (½ cup) sugar
80 ml (⅓ cup) lemon juice
80 ml (⅓ cup) orange juice
finely grated rind of 1 small lemon or orange

FOR THE CUSTARD
500 ml (2 cups) skimmed milk
10 ml (2 tsp) vanilla essence
3 eggs, beaten
80 ml (⅓ cup) sugar

To make the caramel: Mix the sugar, lemon and orange juice and heat gently until the sugar dissolves, then boil rapidly until a golden colour develops. Stir in the rind. Pour into four greased ovenproof ramekins and leave to set.
To make the custard: Mix the milk and vanilla essence together, and bring to the boil. Beat the eggs and sugar together gently and add the boiling milk to this mixture. Whisk until smooth, then pour into greased ramekins – skim off any foam. Place the ramekins in a pan of cold water, so that the water reaches halfway up their sides. Bake at 170 °C for 1½ hours or until the custard is set in the centre. Lift ramekins out of the water and allow to cool in the refrigerator for at least 3–4 hours. Loosen the custard from the edges with a sharp knife. Place a plate on top of each ramekin and gently tip upside down, holding both the plate and the ramekin tightly together. Leave for a few seconds, then give the ramekin a sharp jerk to release the contents. Serve well chilled and garnished with lemon or orange rind.

NUTRITIONAL INFORMATION PER PORTION			
Fat	**Carbohydrate**	**Protein**	**Energy**
(g)	(g)	(g)	(Cal)
4	53	9	278

Quick & Convenient Alternatives
Pick 'n Pay Choice Crème Caramel Dessert
Moirs Crème Caramel – packet
Royal Crème Caramel – packet

Fruity Baked Pudding
SERVES 8–10

Vegetarian ◆ Heart Smart ◆ Diabetic

FOR THE PUDDING
1 x 397-g can fruit cocktail, including juice/syrup
500 ml (2 cups) self-raising flour
8 ml (1½ tsp) bicarbonate of soda
190 ml (¾ cup) sugar
2 eggs, beaten
a pinch of salt

FOR THE SAUCE
1 x 410-g can lite evaporated milk
5 ml (1 tsp) almond/vanilla essence

To make the pudding: Mix all the ingredients together to form a moist, smooth dough. Pour into a large, rectangular, greased, ovenproof dish. Bake at 180 °C for 30 minutes.

To make the sauce: Mix the ingredients and boil for 5 minutes, then pour over the hot pudding just before serving. The pudding can also be served cold, if preferred.

NUTRITIONAL INFORMATION PER PORTION			
Fat (g)	Carbohydrate (g)	Protein (g)	Energy (Cal)
3	50	7	258

Baked Lemon Rice Pudding

SERVES 6–8

Vegetarian ◆ Heart Smart ◆ Diabetic

165 ml (⅔ cup) brown rice
2 eggs, separated
125 ml (½ cup) castor sugar
250 ml (1 cup) self-raising flour
a pinch of salt
5 ml (1 tsp) ground cinnamon
1 lemon, juice and finely grated rind
500 ml (2 cups) skimmed milk

Prepare the rice according to the manufacturer's instructions, and set it aside. Beat the egg-whites until stiff peaks form, then set aside. Beat the egg-yolks and sugar together until smooth, pale yellow and fluffy. Sift the flour, salt and cinnamon together, and set aside. Mix the lemon juice, rind and milk together, and set aside. Now add the flour mixture and the milk mixture, little by little from each one, to the egg-yolk mixture until all the ingredients are well mixed. Mix in the rice and the egg-whites. Pour the mixture into a greased, ovenproof dish and bake at 180 °C for about an hour, until golden brown and well risen. Make a thick syrup by boiling half a cup of sugar, the juice from 1 lemon and half a cup of water in a saucepan. Pour this over the hot, baked pudding. Serve with fat-free custard or low-fat plain yoghurt and drizzled with honey.

NUTRITIONAL INFORMATION PER PORTION			
Fat	Carbohydrate	Protein	Energy
(g)	(g)	(g)	(Cal)
2	43	7	227

Meringue with Toasted Almonds

SERVES 6

Vegetarian ◆ Heart Smart ◆ Diabetic

2 egg-whites
2 ml (½ tsp) cream of tartar
125 ml (½ cup) castor sugar
2 ml (½ tsp) vanilla essence
30 ml (2 tbsp) toasted almonds, chopped

Beat the egg-whites until just foamy, then add the cream of tartar. Continue to beat the mixture until stiff peaks are formed. Now add the sugar a little at a time and beat until glossy. Add the vanilla essence and nuts and beat until the nuts are well distributed. Pipe the meringue mixture onto a lined or non-stick baking sheet and bake at 100 °C for 2½ hours, or until dry. Serve with fruit toppings or custard.

NUTRITIONAL INFORMATION PER PORTION			
Fat (g)	Carbohydrate (g)	Protein (g)	Energy (Cal)
1	17	2	84

Quick & Convenient Alternatives
Pick 'n Pay Foodhall Meringue – mini baskets or rosettes

CHEF'S TIP
Sandwich two meringues together with fat-free, smooth, sweetened cottage cheese and drizzle with a fruit sauce or custard.

Baked Buttermilk Pudding

SERVES 6–8

Vegetarian ◆ Heart Smart ◆ Diabetic

500 ml (2 cups) skimmed milk
250 ml (1 cup) buttermilk
2 eggs, beaten
190 ml (¾ cup) sugar
15 ml (1 tbsp) low-fat margarine
10 ml (2 tsp) vanilla essence
190 ml (¾ cup) self-raising flour

Mix all the ingredients together to form a smooth batter. Pour into a greased or non-stick pie dish. Bake at 180 °C for approximately 45 minutes until golden brown.

NUTRITIONAL INFORMATION PER PORTION			
Fat	Carbohydrate	Protein	Energy
(g)	(g)	(g)	(Cal)
3	40	7	210

DIETICIAN'S TIP

For those with an after-dinner sweet tooth, a cup of Milo or Horlicks, or even hot chocolate made with fat-free milk is a satisfying treat. Add a marshmallow for a touch of decadence.

Crustless Milk Tart

SERVES 6–8

Vegetarian ◆ Heart Smart ◆ Diabetic

1 x 397-g can low-fat condensed milk
2½ condensed milk tins full of water
3 heaped tbsp cornflour
2 eggs, separated
10 ml (2 tsp) vanilla essence

Mix the condensed milk and water, and gently heat in a saucepan. Meanwhile, mix the cornflour to a paste with a little water and add this to the heated milk. Add the beaten egg-yolks and vanilla essence and stir in. Beat the egg-whites until stiff, and fold this into the milk mixture. Pour

NUTRITIONAL INFORMATION PER PORTION			
Fat (g)	Carbohydrate (g)	Protein (g)	Energy (Cal)
2	39	8	195

Quick & Convenient Alternative

Farmers Pride Instant Milk Tart Mix – packet

BAKED GOODS

Cheese & Chive Muffins
MAKES 8–10

Vegetarian ◆ Heart Smart ◆ Diabetic

125 ml (½ cup) whole-wheat flour
125 ml (½ cup) cake flour
3 ml (½ tsp) salt
3 ml (½ tsp) bicarbonate of soda
125 ml (½ cup) skimmed milk
5 ml (1 tsp) sugar
1 large egg, beaten
30 ml (2 tbsp) melted margarine or vegetable oil
5 ml (1 tsp) mustard powder
75 ml (5 tbsp) grated Lichten Blanc/Woolworths
reduced-fat Cheddar cheese
5 ml (1 tsp) dried chives or 15 ml
(1 tbsp) freshly chopped chives

Mix the flour, salt and bicarbonate of soda together. In a separate bowl, mix the milk, sugar and egg. Make a well in the centre of the dry ingredients and add the milk mixture. Using a large spoon, fold the mixture to form a soft dough. Add the additional ingredients to obtain the chosen flavour. Spoon the muffin mixture into a well-greased or non-stick muffin tray. Bake at 200 °C for 20 minutes until the muffins are well risen and golden brown.

NUTRITIONAL INFORMATION PER PORTION			
Fat (g)	Carbohydrate (g)	Protein (g)	Energy (Cal)
4	23	7	158

Overnight Spice Muffins
MAKES 12–14

Vegetarian ◆ Heart Smart ◆ Diabetic

250 ml (1 cup) nutty wheat flour
250 ml (1 cup) cake flour
125 ml (½ cup) soft brown sugar
7 ml (1½ tsp) bicarbonate of soda
a pinch of salt
250 ml (1 cup) skimmed milk
5 ml (1 tsp) vanilla essence
1 egg, beaten
125 ml (½ cup) raisins
5 ml (1 tsp) cinnamon, ground
2 ml (½ tsp) nutmeg, ground
2 ml (½ tsp) mixed spice, ground

Mix together all the ingredients to form a moist dough. Cover and leave in the refrigerator overnight. Spoon the dough into a greased muffin tray until the individual cups are two thirds full. Bake for 15–20 minutes at 200 °C until well risen. Allow to cool in the tray for 2 minutes, then turn out onto a wire rack.

NUTRITIONAL INFORMATION PER PORTION			
Fat (g)	Carbohydrate (g)	Protein (g)	Energy (Cal)
2	74	10	361

Quick & Convenient Alternative
Pillsbury Banana Nut Muffin Mix – packet

Mealie Bread

SERVES 8–10

Vegetarian ◆ Heart Smart ◆ Diabetic

250 ml (1 cup) mealie meel
250 ml (1 cup) flour
125 ml (½ cup) sugar
15 ml (1 tbsp) baking powder
5 ml (1 tsp) salt
250 ml (1 cup) skimmed milk
3 eggs, beaten
1 x 410 g-can sweetcorn

Mix together all the dry ingredients in a mixing bowl. In a separate bowl, mix together all the liquid ingredients. Add the liquid mixture to the dry ingredients and mix well to form a smooth dough. Pour into a greased glass bowl and steam, covered, over a pot of boiling water for about 1½ hours, or until cooked. This bread is delicious served with a braai.

NUTRITIONAL INFORMATION PER PORTION			
Fat (g)	Carbohydrate (g)	Protein (g)	Energy (Cal)
2	44	6	220

Italian Biscotti

MAKES ABOUT 80 THIN BARS

Heart Smart ◆ Diabetic

100 g (¼ cup) toasted almonds
3 egg-whites
250 ml (1 cup) castor sugar
250 ml (1 cup) cake flour

Mix all the ingredients together, pour the dough into a loaf tin prepared with Spray and Cook, and bake at 140 °C for 15–20 minutes or until the dough is just brown. Cool, cut into thin slices of about 2 mm thick, then return to the oven until crisp and browned.

NUTRITIONAL INFORMATION PER PORTION			
Fat (g)	Carbohydrate (g)	Protein (g)	Energy (Cal)
3	12	2	84

Quick & Convenient Alternative
Woolworths Italian Biscotti

Lager Loaf
SERVES 8–10

Vegetarian ◆ Heart Smart ◆ Diabetic

500 g (3¼ cups) self-raising flour
5 ml (1 tsp) salt
340 ml (1 can) beer (lager)

Mix together all the ingredients to form a moist, firm dough. Pour into a greased loaf pan and bake at 180 °C for 1 hour. Serve hot.

NUTRITIONAL INFORMATION PER PORTION			
Fat (g)	Carbohydrate (g)	Protein (g)	Energy (Cal)
1	41	6	212

Quick & Convenient Alternative
Golden Cloud Cape-Style Bread Mix – packet

Date & Bran Muffins
MAKES 16–18

Vegetarian ◆ Heart Smart ◆ Diabetic

1 x 250 g-block (¾ cup) dates,
pitted and finely chopped
125 ml (½ cup) raisins
250 ml (1 cup) boiling water
5 ml (1 tsp) bicarbonate of soda
750 ml (3 cups) nutty wheat flour
60 ml (¼ cup) soft brown sugar
5 ml (1 tsp) bicarbonate of soda, extra
1 egg, beaten
250 ml (1 cup) buttermilk
5 ml (1 tsp) vanilla essence

Mix the dates and raisins with the boiling water and 1 tsp bicarbonate of soda, and set aside to soak. Mix together the flour, sugar and 1 tsp bicarbonate of soda in a mixing bowl. Beat together the egg, buttermilk and vanilla essence, and add this to the date mixture. Add the liquid mixture to the dry ingredients, and mix lightly with a knife until a moist dough is formed – do not overmix. Spoon the dough into a greased muffin tray, until the individual cups are each two thirds full. Bake for 15–20 minutes at 200 °C until well risen. Allow to cool in the tray for 2 minutes, then turn the muffins out onto a wire rack.

NUTRITIONAL INFORMATION PER PORTION			
Fat (g)	Carbohydrate (g)	Protein (g)	Energy (Cal)
2	71	11	361

Quick & Convenient Alternative
Weigh-less Bran Muffin Dough – frozen

Herb Scones
MAKES 10–12

Vegetarian ◆ Heart Smart ◆ Diabetic

375 ml (1½ cups) flour,
whole-wheat or plain
3 ml (½ tsp) salt
3 ml (½ tsp) bicarbonate of soda
10 ml (2 tsp) garlic and herb seasoning
5 ml (1 tsp) freshly chopped rosemary
5 ml (1 tsp) freshly chopped parsley
5 ml (1 tsp) freshly chopped thyme
3 ml (½ tsp) paprika
200 ml (¾ cup) cultured buttermilk or
fat-free plain yoghurt
milk to glaze

Mix together the flour, salt and bicarbonate of soda. Add the herbs and
the paprika. Make a well in the centre of the dry ingredients and pour
in the buttermilk or yoghurt. Mix to form a firm dough. Turn the dough
out onto a lightly floured surface, and knead lightly to remove any cracks.
Roll out to a thickness of about 2 cm and cut into rounds. Brush the
tops with milk and place the scones on a non-stick baking sheet. Bake
for 20 minutes at 200 °C until well risen and golden brown. Serve warm
with cottage cheese.

NUTRITIONAL INFORMATION PER PORTION			
Fat	Carbohydrate	Protein	Energy
(g)	(g)	(g)	(Cal)
1	36	4	178

Nutty Fruit Cake

SERVES 10–12

Vegetarian ◆ Heart Smart ◆ Diabetic

250 ml (1 cup) dates, pitted
300 ml (1¼ cups) water
450 g (1½ cups) fruit mix
350 ml (1¼ cups) whole-wheat flour
15 ml (1 tbsp) baking powder
5 ml (1 tsp) mixed spice
60 ml (4 tbsp) orange juice
30 g (2 tbsp) ground almonds
grated rind of 1 orange/lemon
a pinch of salt
2 capfuls of brandy (optional)

In a suacepan, add the dates to the water and gently bring to the boil. Mash the dates and add all the other ingredients. Mix well. Spoon the mixture into a greased and lightly floured loaf tin and bake at 160 °C for 1½ hours. Pour brandy over (if using) while the cake is still hot.

NUTRITIONAL INFORMATION PER PORTION			
Fat	**Carbohydrate**	**Protein**	**Energy**
(g)	(g)	(g)	(Cal)
2	50	3	239

Cheese & Garlic Braai Bread

SERVES 8–10

Vegetarian ◆ Heart Smart ◆ Diabetic

12 fresh chives, washed and chopped
5 cloves garlic, peeled and crushed
1 tub (250 g) fat-free cream cheese or cottage cheese
salt and freshly ground pepper to taste
a splash of Tabasco sauce (optional)
1 French loaf, cut into slices diagonally
(not all the way through)

Mix together the chives, garlic and cream cheese. Season to taste. Spread the mixture onto one side of each slice of bread. Wrap in tinfoil. Bake at 180 °C for 15 minutes or over hot coals until heated through.

NUTRITIONAL INFORMATION PER PORTION			
Fat (g)	Carbohydrate (g)	Protein (g)	Energy (Cal)
1	11	5	69

DIETICIAN'S TIPS

To make some great low-fat braai snacks:
Toss diced red, yellow, and green peppers in fresh garlic and seasoning and braai on the grid. Do the same with mushrooms, and eat them straight off the braai grid.

DRESSINGS, SAUCES & MARINADES

Thousand Islands Dressing
MAKES ABOUT 1 CUP

Vegetarian ◆ Heart Smart ◆ Diabetic

250 ml (1 cup) cultured buttermilk
15 ml (1 tbsp) tomato sauce
15 ml (1 tbsp) Trim mayonnaise
15 ml (1 tbsp) fruit chutney
2–5 drops Tabasco sauce
5 ml (1 tsp) mustard powder
1 clove garlic, peeled and crushed

Mix all the ingredients and blend together until smooth. Serve well chilled. Store in a closed bottle in the refrigerator.

NUTRITIONAL INFORMATION PER PORTION			
Fat (g)	**Carbohydrate** (g)	**Protein** (g)	**Energy** (Cal)
2	4	2	38

Quick & Convenient Alternatives
Royco Lite Creamy Thousand Islands Dressing
Heinz Fat-free Thousand Islands Dressing

Barbecue Braai Sauce

SERVES 4

Vegetarian ◆ Heart Smart ◆ Diabetic

125 ml (½ cup) tomato sauce
30 ml (2 tbsp) Worcestershire sauce
1 clove garlic, peeled and crushed
a pinch of salt
30 ml (2 tbsp) sticky brown sugar
15 ml (1 tbsp) vinegar
a pinch of mustard

Mix all the ingredients together, and boil for 5 minutes. Allow to cool and store in the refrigerator. This sauce is particularly good as a basting sauce for kebabs, or as a relish.

NUTRITIONAL INFORMATION PER PORTION			
Fat	**Carbohydrate**	**Protein**	**Energy**
(g)	(g)	(g)	(Cal)
trace	8	1	54

Quick & Convenient Alternatives
Steers Steakmaker Braai Sauce
Heinz BBQ Cajun Style Sauce
Knorr Spare Rib Braai Sauce

CHEF'S TIP
For a braai, wrap diced butternut or pumpkin in foil with a little garlic, salt and pepper, and bake directly on the coals until soft.

Nam Jin Dressing

SERVES 4

Heart Smart ◆ Diabetic

1 clove garlic, peeled and crushed
2–3 fresh coriander leaves, chopped
3 ml (½ tsp) salt
2 fresh chillies, crushed
15 ml (1 tbsp) sugar
15 ml (1 tbsp) Thai fish sauce
15 ml (1 tbsp) lime juice
30 ml (2 tbsp) balsamic vinegar
1 pickled onion, grated

Blend all the ingredients together and store in a closed bottle in the refrigerator.

NUTRITIONAL INFORMATION PER PORTION			
Fat (g)	Carbohydrate (g)	Protein (g)	Energy (Cal)
3	6	2	56

Lemon & Sun-Dried Tomato Dressing

SERVES 4–6

Vegetarian ◆ Heart Smart ◆ Diabetic

1 onion, peeled and finely chopped
15 ml (1 tbsp) freshly chopped thyme
80 ml (⅓ cup) lemon juice
80 ml (⅓ cup) sun-dried tomatoes, chopped
80 ml (⅓ cup) pine nuts, roasted
15 ml (1 tbsp) sugar

Mix all the ingredients together, and blend in a liquidizer until smooth. Serve well chilled and store in the refrigerator.

NUTRITIONAL INFORMATION PER PORTION			
Fat (g)	Carbohydrate (g)	Protein (g)	Energy (Cal)
0	4	1	19

Sweet & Sour Dressing
SERVES 4

Vegetarian ◆ Heart Smart ◆ Diabetic

5 ml (1 tsp) cornflour
125 ml (½ cup) orange juice
2 slices fresh pineapple, finely chopped
1 clove garlic, peeled and crushed
2 cm root ginger, peeled and finely grated
15 ml (1 tbsp) soy sauce
1 pickled onion, finely chopped
2 gherkins, finely chopped

Mix the cornflour to a paste with a little water. Boil the orange juice, then add the cornflour paste. Heat until the mixture thickens. Add to the other ingredients and blend in a liquidizer until smooth. Store in a closed bottle in the refrigerator.

NUTRITIONAL INFORMATION PER PORTION			
Fat (g)	Carbohydrate (g)	Protein (g)	Energy (Cal)
trace	7	1	30

Satay Sauce
SERVES 4

Vegetarian ◆ Diabetic

50 g (3–4 tbsp) peanut butter
1 clove garlic, peeled and crushed
2.5 cm root ginger, peeled and finely grated
30 ml (2 tbsp) soy sauce
30 ml (2 tbsp) honey
125 ml (½ cup) coconut milk
1 lemon, juice only
1 fresh chilli, minced

Mix all the ingredients and bring the mixture to the boil, then reduce heat and simmer for 8 minutes. The sauce will thicken slightly. Allow to cool a little before serving. Serve with chicken pieces.

NUTRITIONAL INFORMATION PER PORTION			
Fat	Carbohydrate	Protein	Energy
(g)	(g)	(g)	(Cal)
8	19	5	159

Tartare Sauce
MAKES ABOUT 1 CUP

Vegetarian ◆ Heart Smart ◆ Diabetic

90 ml (⅔ cup) fat-free plain yoghurt
60 ml (¼ cup) Trim mayonnaise
2 large gherkins, chopped
half an onion, peeled and finely grated
5 ml (1 tsp) freshly chopped parsley
15 ml (1 tbsp) freshly chopped basil
1–2 drops Tabasco sauce

Mix all the ingredients together thoroughly and serve chilled. This is particularly good with fish.

NUTRITIONAL INFORMATION PER PORTION			
Fat (g)	Carbohydrate (g)	Protein (g)	Energy (Cal)
3	4	2	49

Indian Tikka Sauce
SERVES 2–4

Vegetarian ◆ Heart Smart ◆ Diabetic

1 onion, peeled and sliced
30 ml (2 tbsp) tomato purée
10 ml (2 tsp) freshly grated ginger
2 cloves garlic, peeled and crushed
15 ml (1 tbsp) ground coriander
15 ml (1 tbsp) ground cumin
1 fresh chilli, chopped
125 ml (½ cup) fat-free plain yoghurt
5 ml (1 tsp) stock powder or Aromat
45 ml (3 tbsp) lemon juice

Blend all the ingredients together in a liquidizer until smooth. Serve with chicken salad as a starter or main course.

NUTRITIONAL INFORMATION PER PORTION			
Fat (g)	Carbohydrate (g)	Protein (g)	Energy (Cal)
trace	7	3	40

Honey & Mustard Sauce
MAKES ABOUT 1½ CUPS

Heart Smart ◆ Diabetic

4–6 spring onions, sliced
15 ml (1 tbsp) freshly chopped thyme
1 clove garlic, peeled and crushed
375 ml (1½ cups) chicken stock
60 ml (4 tbsp) prepared Dijon mustard
30 ml (2 tbsp) honey
15 ml (1 tbsp) cornflour

Cook the onion, thyme and garlic in a little stock until tender. Add the mustard, honey and remaining stock. Mix the cornflour to a smooth paste with a little water, then add to the sauce. Cook until the sauce thickens. This is delicious with chicken or as a hot salad dressing.

NUTRITIONAL INFORMATION PER PORTION			
Fat	**Carbohydrate**	**Protein**	**Energy**
(g)	(g)	(g)	(Cal)
1	11	1	53

Quick & Convenient Alternatives
Woolworths Honey & Mustard Grill & Bake Sauce – ready-made
Walnut Ridge Creamy Honey & Mustard Unbelievable Chicken Sauce – ready-made

DIETICIAN'S TIP
It is a fallacy that honey is better for you than sugar – honey does contain trace amounts of certain minerals, but not enough to warrant even a mention in terms of nutritional value.

Cold Savoury Sauce for Chicken
SERVES 4

Vegetarian ◆ Heart Smart ◆ Diabetic

1 onion, peeled and chopped
1 green pepper, seeded and chopped
15 ml (1 tbsp) tomato purée
a pinch each of cayenne pepper, nutmeg and paprika
15 ml (1 tbsp) curry powder
60 ml (4 tbsp) red wine
30 ml (2 tbsp) apricot jam
30 ml (2 tbsp) Trim mayonnaise
175 ml (1 small tub) fat-free plain yoghurt

Mix all the ingredients, except the mayonnaise and yoghurt, and bring to the boil. Reduce the heat and simmer for 5 minutes. Allow to cool. Add the mayonnaise and yoghurt. Blend until smooth and serve with chicken.

NUTRITIONAL INFORMATION PER PORTION			
Fat (g)	Carbohydrate (g)	Protein (g)	Energy (Cal)
2	18	4	113

Fat-Free Savoury White Sauce
MAKES ABOUT 2 CUPS

Vegetarian ◆ Heart Smart ◆ Diabetic

500 ml (2 cups) skimmed milk
1 small onion, peeled and chopped
a pinch of freshly chopped thyme
45 ml (3 tbsp) cornflour
15 ml (1 tbsp) stock powder
10 ml (2 tsp) mustard powder

Mix the milk, onion and thyme together, and bring to the boil. Mix the cornflour, stock powder and mustard powder to a smooth, thin paste with a little water. Add this to the boiled milk mixture and stir, while allowing the sauce to thicken.

NUTRITIONAL INFORMATION PER PORTION			
Fat (g)	Carbohydrate (g)	Protein (g)	Energy (Cal)
trace	7	3	42

Quick & Convenient Alternatives
Royco Cheese, Wild Mushroom or White Sauce – packet
Pick 'n Pay Choice Fresh Cheese or Mushroom Sauce – ready-made

---

CHEF'S TIPS
To make a cheese sauce: *Add 5 ml (1 tsp) dried Parmesan cheese once the sauce has thickened.*
To make a mushroom sauce: *Add 35 g (½ cup) sliced mushrooms to the milk and onion mixture.*
To make a herb sauce: *Add 50 ml (¼ cup) freshly chopped tarragon – for chicken and/or egg dishes.*
Add 50 ml (¼ cup) freshly chopped chives – for pasta dishes.
Add 50 ml (¼ cup) freshly chopped basil – for meat, and cheese/tomato dishes.

Napoletana Sauce

SERVES 4

Vegetarian ◆ Heart Smart ◆ Diabetic

1 onion, peeled and chopped
1 small green pepper, seeded and chopped
3 ripe tomatoes, chopped
1 clove garlic, crushed
125 ml (½ cup) freshly chopped parsley
15 ml (1 tbsp) sugar
25 ml (2 tbsp) paprika
250 ml (1 cup) wine
15 ml (1tbsp) stock powder

Mix all the ingredients together and bring to the boil, then simmer for 20 minutes. Serve with pasta or add to bolognaise.

NUTRITIONAL INFORMATION PER PORTION			
Fat (g)	Carbohydrate (g)	Protein (g)	Energy (Cal)
trace	10	2	90

Lemon & Garlic Marinade for Chicken or Fish

SERVES 4

Vegetarian ◆ Heart Smart ◆ Diabetic

1 orange, juice and finely grated rind
1 lemon, juice and finely grated rind
4 cloves garlic, peeled and crushed
1 red chilli, finely chopped or minced
15 ml (1 tbsp) freshly chopped thyme

Blend all the ingredients together. Pour over chicken or fish strips or fillets. Cover and marinate for 2–3 hours in the refrigerator. Cook the chicken or fish as usual thereafter.

To use the marinade as a sauce: Mix 2 tsp cornflour with a little water to form a smooth, thin paste, whilst bringing the marinade mixture to the boil. Add the cornflour to the boiling marinade and stir until the mixture thickens. Serve immediately with seasonal vegetables.

NUTRITIONAL INFORMATION PER PORTION			
Fat (g)	Carbohydrate (g)	Protein (g)	Energy (Cal)
trace	6	1	26

Teriyaki Marinade
SERVES 4

Vegetarian ◆ Heart Smart ◆ Diabetic

4 cloves garlic, peeled and crushed
30 ml (2 tbsp) soft brown sugar
60 ml (¼ cup) soy sauce
60 ml (¼ cup) sherry
30 ml (2 tbsp) freshly grated root ginger

Mix all the ingredients together, and blend thoroughly. Marinate meat strips overnight in the refrigerator in a covered container. Cook the meat as usual thereafter.

NUTRITIONAL INFORMATION PER PORTION			
Fat (g)	Carbohydrate (g)	Protein (g)	Energy (Cal)
0	10	2	56

Mango & Mint Relish

SERVES 4–6

Vegetarian ◆ Heart Smart ◆ Diabetic

1 small onion, peeled and finely chopped
2 medium-sized mangoes, chopped
5 ml (1 tsp) brown sugar
15 ml (1 tbsp) balsamic vinegar
15 ml (1 tbsp) freshly chopped mint leaves

Mix the chopped onion and mango, and cook over low heat for about 5 minutes. Add the sugar and the vinegar and simmer for a further 10 minutes. Add the mint and stir well. Chill thoroughly and serve as an accompaniment to chicken, lamb or Mexican dishes.

NUTRITIONAL INFORMATION PER PORTION			
Fat (g)	Carbohydrate (g)	Protein (g)	Energy (Cal)
trace	19	1	72

Easy Apricot Chutney

MAKES ABOUT 2 CUPS

Vegetarian ◆ Heart Smart ◆ Diabetic

125 ml (½ cup) dried apricots
125 ml (½ cup) brown vinegar
30 ml (2 tbsp) water
60 ml (¼ cup) raisins
125 ml (½ cup) fresh dates, stoned and chopped
1 large apple, cored and coarsely chopped
3 cloves garlic, peeled and crushed
1 medium onion, peeled and chopped
30 ml (2 tbsp) soft brown sugar
a pinch each of ground ginger,
cinnamon and cayenne pepper
salt and coarsely ground black pepper to taste

Soak the apricots in the vinegar and water overnight. Mix with all the other ingredients, then blend in a liquidizer until an even, but chunky consistency is reached. Pour the chutney into a sterilised bottle and store in the refrigerator.

NUTRITIONAL INFORMATION PER PORTION			
Fat (g)	Carbohydrate (g)	Protein (g)	Energy (Cal)
trace	18	1	75

CHEF'S TIP
This apricot chutney makes a wonderful accompaniment to bobotie and curries, and can also be spread on sandwiches.

CHAPTER FOUR

Restaurant Guide

GENERAL GUIDELINES TO FOLLOW
WHEN DINING OUT

Due to increased consumer awareness of low-fat food options, most restaurants are starting to provide more health-conscious menu items and introducing more flexibility in terms of their food preparation. In the course of researching and compiling the list of restaurants to be found in this chapter I have, in general, found both restaurant managers and owners to be extremely obliging and very keen to help give patrons whatever they request.

When you are dining out, the most important thing to remember is that you are the client. As you are paying for the meal, you have the right to ask for food to be prepared freshly according to your particular requirements. Therefore, even though a menu may state that vegetables are stir-fried, you should be able to order your vegetables steamed. You should also be able to order foods that may not appear on the menu. If a menu lists 'English Breakfast' or 'Continental Breakfast', it should not mean that patrons cannot order poached eggs on unbuttered toast with grilled or fresh tomato, for instance. Always ask whether your food may be grilled, steamed or baked without fat, even if these cooking options are not given on the menu. Sometimes you may need to explain in detail what you mean when asking for no fat to be used, so specify that, for example, no oil, margarine, butter or cream is to be used.

If it seems that your particular requirements cannot be met, it may be that you are asking the wrong person. In my experience waitrons are, in general, often less likely to be accommodating than restaurant managers or owners. Waitrons usually work under considerable and various pressures. It may, thus, be quicker and easier for them to say that low-fat milk is not available, rather than to go and check. Faced with the wrath of a stressed chef, it may be much easier to say that baked potatoes are not served. Now is the time for customers to use their skills of persuasion, however, and, if necessary, speak to the manager personally.

In certain social situations, you may find it rather awkward to order specially prepared foods. If you want to avoid drawing attention to your individual requirements, either telephone ahead to place your order, or order your food like everyone else and, a few moments later, subtly go and change your order on your way to the bathroom. If someone notices and comments on your requests, my advice is not to give weight loss as the reason for your special requirements. In my experience, a recent stomach upset, allergy or high blood cholesterol problem may far more readily be accepted as an explanation.

If you plan to have alcohol with your meal, remember to count alcohol as a carbohydrate portion. Compensate by omitting some of the carbohydrates you would otherwise have eaten. To enjoy a guilt-free two or three glasses of wine, I suggest ordering a plain salad as a starter, followed by ostrich steak, grilled fish or calamari with fresh lemon and steamed vegetables, rounded off with fresh fruit salad and coffee.

RECOMMENDED STARTERS

If you want to avoid overindulgence it is often useful to order two or more starters rather than a main course, or to share a main dish with one or more fellow diners. If your companions have ordered starters and you prefer only having one course, it is a good idea not to sit idly watching others eat while you wait for them to reach the main course. If you anticipate a long wait, fill up on a slice of bread or a plain salad. Watching others eat while you are hungry is torture, and this may simply lead you to overeat when your food finally arrives.

The following suggestions are good options for starters:

❖ Choose a salad with no dressing or mayonnaise – use vinegar or lemon juice – and avoid bacon, croûtons and cheeses. Opt for smoked chicken, smoked salmon, tuna or seafood, or a Greek salad. A simple French salad usually has the lowest fat content and is ideal, especially if you are planning to have protein (meat or cheese) as part of your main dish.

❖ Stock-based soups or thick vegetable soups with no cream garnish

❖ Fresh bread with smoked salmon or tzatziki

❖ Fruit cocktails, melon balls or fruit platters

- Tasty mussels or calamari in a wine or tomato-based sauce, or oysters
- Meze consisting of tzatziki, dolmades, olives, hummus and pita bread
- Grilled calamari or other seafood basted with lemon juice only
- Spinach and feta or ricotta in phyllo pastry (for example, spanakopitka)

RECOMMENDED MAIN DISHES

In general, it is a safer option to order plain separate food items, such as grilled fish, baked potato and steamed vegetables, rather than combination dishes such as lasagne, curries, casseroles or moussaka. Combination dishes are often made with sauces with hidden fats that can result in a meal with a surprisingly high fat content.

- Pastas with tomato-based sauce rather than a cream, pesto or cheese-based sauce. It is often advisable to order the pasta and sauce separately – if the sauce looks too oily, you can use just a little and fill up on the pasta. Better still – ask for no oil or cream and order pasta with chicken, salmon, ham, seafood, mushrooms, vegetables, herbs, garlic, chilli, etc. For example, one of my favourite pasta dishes contains spinach, garlic, tomato, ham, courgette and cream – and it is just as delicious when I order it without oil or cream. For a strong cheese flavour, add one teaspoon of Parmesan cheese.
- Order your pizza with half the cheese or even with no cheese – have toppings like tomato (fresh or sun-dried), onion, green pepper, garlic, chilli, mushroom, asparagus, ham, pineapple, banana, chicken, peppadews, a sprinkling of feta, spinach, olives, egg, tuna, anchovies, or seafood – avoid salami, bacon, sausage, mince and cheese. A sprinkling of feta used with the above fillings – and no mozzarella – is very tasty. Although mozzarella and feta have similar fat contents, you would need a lot less feta to get the same cheesy flavour, as mozzarella is a fairly bland cheese. Order a pizza with a thin base, as a thick base may be too dry without any cheese. If you are ordering pita bread, ask for very little oil or no oil to be added. Herb bread may be a better choice, as the garlic paste used in many restaurants is oil-based. Many pizza restaurants baste the

pizza with oil as it comes out of the oven to keep it from drying out, so remember to ask for no oil basting. St Elmo's restaurants (*see* pages 199 and 200) have even allowed for this request to be accommodated on their computer system with your order.

❖ If you are ordering steak, have it plain or with a barbecue sauce (no creamy sauces) and choose a fillet, sirloin or T-bone rather than a rump. Remember – eat only your allowed quota of protein (your dog will enjoy the rest!). It is often a good idea to order the ladies' portion. If there is no option, cut your steak in half as soon as it is placed in front of you, and send half back to be put straight into a doggy bag. Resist the habit – usually acquired in childhood – of eating everything on your plate. Instead of gravy, have mint sauce or jelly with lamb, mustard or horseradish with beef, and apple sauce with pork. Avoid the Cordon Bleus and Schnitzels, as these are both high-fat options.

❖ Few people regularly prepare venison or ostrich at home, so these are great when you are dining out and want to try something new. Watch out for creamy sauces, though. Both of these meats are complemented by strong flavours such as mustard, black pepper or barbecue sauce.

❖ Order grilled or poached fish rather than fish prepared in a batter. Select types of fish that are lower in fat, like hake, kabeljou, sole and kingklip, for instance. Avoid oily fish like salmon, mackerel, snoek and butterfish. Sushi has become a popular low-fat choice.

❖ Grilled seafood is also a good option – without the mayonnaise or tartare sauce. Ask for your crayfish or prawns to be boiled or grilled with no fat, and simply use a squeeze of fresh lemon.

❖ Vegetarian meal options are often fried or covered in cheese sauces, so check with your waitron.

❖ Order steamed rice, baked potatoes (with no butter or sour cream – most restaurants do have cottage cheese), or steamed vegetables instead of chips, fried rice or roast potatoes.

RECOMMENDED DESSERTS OR NIGHTCAPS

Eating a peppermint is often an easy way of dealing with a desire for something sweet after dinner, so grab one on your way to the bathroom while everyone else is ordering dessert. If you feel like just a taste of cheesecake, for example, do not be tempted to order a whole slice. Rather ask a friend for a taste of his or hers, or even share a pudding with one or two fellow diners. Your wallets and waistlines will benefit.

- ❖ Cappuccino with a milk froth (preferably used skimmed milk or low-fat milk)
- ❖ Crème caramel
- ❖ Frozen yoghurt
- ❖ Fruit salad with yoghurt
- ❖ Sorbet or low-fat ice-cream
- ❖ Fruit mousse
- ❖ Strawberries and meringues
- ❖ Pears in red wine
- ❖ A dry port or sherry and fresh fruit (avoid creamy liqueurs)
- ❖ If you are having cheese and biscuits, choose a soft goat's cheese or feta rather than a hard cheese and have it on a plain cracker such as Pro-Vita rather than a savoury cracker.

RECOMMENDED BREAKFASTS

The following options may not necessarily appear on the menu, but there is no reason why the dishes cannot be prepared for you.

- ❖ Two poached or boiled eggs on toast (using no margarine or butter) with a grilled or fresh tomato. It is fine using condiments such as tomato sauce, Worcestershire sauce and HP Sauce. I often ask for scrambled eggs on toast, and ask for as little fat as possible to be used in scrambling the eggs. In fact, if a restaurant can microwave the eggs or if they use a non-stick frying pan, no fat is needed. Many restaurants add cream to their scrambled-egg mixture – so find out.
- ❖ Anchovy toast (using no margarine or butter) – this is very nice topped with fresh slices of tomato or herbs
- ❖ Mashed banana on toast
- ❖ A bran muffin – plain or with jam
- ❖ Flapjacks or crumpets with syrup
- ❖ Fruit salad – plain or with yoghurt
- ❖ Toast with jam or marmalade (using no margarine)
- ❖ To drink, order fruit juice, tea or coffee with fat-free or low-fat milk. If the restaurant does not have low-fat milk, avoid cappuccino, café latté and other milky hot drinks.

RECOMMENDED TAKE-AWAYS
OR LIGHT MEALS

❖ A hamburger with no sauce – except tomato, barbecue or chilli sauce. Do not order chips or cheese. If you have the option of choosing a chicken patty, do so – especially if it is flame grilled. Always remember to ask for the patty to be flame grilled using no fat – restaurants often add fat before or during the flame-grilling process. A vegetarian burger may, in fact, be higher in fat than a regular beef burger, so unless you are vegetarian, it may not be a wise choice.

❖ Soup (as long as it is not a cream-based variety) and a bread roll

❖ A baked potato with cottage cheese or tuna or chicken (adding no mayonnaise)

❖ A sandwich (made using a roll, bread, pita or a bagel) with beef or ham and mustard (no processed meats), or avocado, or cottage cheese, or chicken, or tuna with salad and pickles (adding no margarine or mayonnaise)

❖ A chicken, tuna, smoked salmon or health salad with no dressing and a pita bread or roll or two slices of bread

❖ Avoid quiches, as the ingredients used in the pastry and filling usually result in a very high fat intake – often even more than pizza.

❖ If you order something like crumbed chicken or fried fish, you can reduce the fat content by removing the batter in which it has been prepared and setting it aside.

NATIONWIDE RESTAURANT GUIDE

In the following section, I have tried to include as wide a range of restaurants as possible, listed in alphabetical order – obviously some excellent restaurants have had to be omitted to prevent this list becoming endless. If the particular restaurant you are visiting does not appear on the list given here, try to locate the entries for a similar kind of restaurant. For example, if you are dining at a restaurant like Panarottis, you may be able to use the menu guide of a similar restaurant, like St Elmo's.

For the purposes of this compilation, wherever possible, an attempt has been made to identify the fat content of various menu items. When this has not been possible, the items containing less fat have been identified. Note that this does not necessarily mean that these are low-fat items.

Also, where it has been advised that you ask a restaurant to prepare your food in a way not normally available on the menu, please be aware that this may not always be possible. So, for example, if you would like to order a toasted chicken mayonnaise sandwich without mayonnaise, this may not be possible at every restaurant, but it is worth asking for.

CANTINA TEQUILA

Mexican cuisine has three main staples: tortillas, fried beans and chilli peppers. Tortillas are cooked on griddles, so they are low in fat. The beans – provided they are boiled only – are an excellent low-fat source of fibre. Chilli peppers also have many healthy qualities due to their high vitamin and mineral content. Therefore, it is possible to order tasty (or fiery!), yet low-fat food from Mexican restaurants. Enjoy plenty of salsa, but avoid the guacamole and sour cream.

Starters
❖ A salad (without dressing) is your best option as a starter course. Go for the Cantina Salad, Calamari Salad or Salad Señorita (without bacon or croûtons).

Main Meals
❖ Burritos – rolled Mexican-style pancakes – topped with salsa (without the cheese) and filled with beef, chicken or vegetables are a tasty treat.
❖ Fajitas (soft flour pancakes with various fillings) are one of the house favourites – as well as being the dietician's favourite.
❖ The 200 g Ranchero Steak or Señorita Steak with rice, tortilla and salad are good choices.
❖ If you are ordering the Poblano Chicken, ask for extra salsa and no creamy green pepper sauce. The Mexican sosaties are also a good choice, especially as you can take one sosatie home to have for dinner the following day.
❖ Grilled seafood is always great, but ask for salsa and fresh lemon instead of butter sauces.

Desserts
❖ The Fruit Brulée has a fairly low fat content.

FISHMONGER

There are more than twenty Fishmonger restaurants nationwide offering Mediterranean seafood.

Starters

❖ The Meze platters can be ordered as starters or main courses, or can be shared. Ask for the squid heads to be grilled and served without lemon butter. Leave out the haloumi and rissoles.

❖ The Mussels Portuguese are a tasty tomato-based mussel dish. If you are ordering the sardines, ask for them to be grilled and to be served without any dressing.

❖ The Calamari starter can be ordered grilled without lemon butter, and the oysters are a healthy, low-fat option.

❖ Check to see whether or not the Soup of the Day is cream-based, otherwise this is a filling, warm starter.

❖ Choose the Greek, Italian or French salad and ask for no dressing – balsamic vinegar should be available.

Main Courses

❖ Ask for all shellfish, calamari and fish to be dry-grilled in the oven and to be served without the lemon butter basting.

❖ Choose the boiled potatoes rather than the chips, and choose the vegetables of the day without sauces.

❖ Pita breads or fresh rolls are also available.

❖ Avoid the Seafood Casserole and the various curries, as they are all cream-based.

Desserts

❖ Share the Crème Brulée with a friend, and order coffee.

J.B. RIVERS
Hyde Park Corner, Johannesburg
Claremont, Cape Town

J.B. Rivers can be described as a 'café and cocktail saloon' and you will find the taste of New Orleans-style spicy Cajun foods, many of which are suitable for diners looking for low-fat meals.

Breakfasts

All breakfasts are served with a glass of fresh fruit juice and tea or coffee. You are also treated to a choice of either skimmed or full-cream milk.

❖ The Light and Healthy or Ladybird breakfasts are both tasty options. Remember to ask for no cream to be added to your scrambled egg if you are ordering the Ladybird. Although the tomato is grilled, the mushrooms are fried in butter, so ask for these to be grilled also.

❖ A bran muffin or scone with preserves is another good choice for breakfast or even as a snack or light meal.

Light Meals

❖ Choose anchovy toast with no butter, or a toasted ham and tomato sandwich, also with no butter.

Salads

All the salads, except the seafood salad can be ordered without dressing. They are all accompanied by bread rolls, so they make complete meals.

❖ Order JB's Health Salad with the sweet soya and lemon juice dressing (with no croûtons) or Balbosa Island Green Salad (without the dressing and croûtons).

❖ The Howlin' Wolf's Chicken Salad or the Laguna Beach Salmon Salad are both delicious and very satisfying low-fat meals.

Open Sandwiches

Remember to ask for no butter to be used on the bread, and also for no mayonnaise or dressings.

❖ The Right Stuff is the right low-fat option, filled with good stuff and containing no hidden traps.

❖ The Hot Pastrami, Rare Roast Beef and Cajun Chicken Treat are also good options, and even the Smoked Salmon Bagel is great if ordered with cottage cheese instead of cream cheese.

Grills and Specialities

J.B. Rivers has made a real effort for low-fat diners and instead of stir-fried vegetables you can order a side salad.

❖ In this section Rocco's Baked Potato springs to mind (and not to thighs) when ordered without the bacon bits and sour cream.

- BB King's Cajun Chicken can be ordered grilled with plain yellow rice or a baked potato and a side salad.
- The same applies to the Bayou Catch of the Day, JB's Steak on French and Riverland Café Blackened Fillet.
- The Seafood Sampler is basically a tomato-based seafood casserole served on pasta, and can be safely sampled.
- The vegetable Memphis Slim Fajita is, believe it or not, a slim option – even with the refried beans (which are actually boiled).
- If you are ordering the chicken or beef Fajita, ask for it to be grilled and served without any barbecue sauce.

Desserts
- Fresh fruit salad with yoghurt, or Milo, hot chocolate or Horlicks made with skimmed milk will satisfy that sweet tooth.
- You may like to choose a cocktail which is not cream-based, or try some speciality coffee.

KEGS

These pubs specialize in traditional English pub fare, which, believe it or not, includes several great low-fat options. The portions are generous, so remember to take extras home as doggy bags to be enjoyed the next day. All vegetarian options (i. e. no meat, chicken or fish) are marked with a 'V'.

Starters
- Bruschetta without butter is a filling starter, and it can even serve as a main meal if ordered with a salad.

Salads
- All salad dressings are supplied separately, so they can easily be avoided. Try the Greek, Smoked Chicken or Peppered Beef Salad.

Lighter Fare
- Ask for the Steak Sandwich to be dry-grilled, or order the Club Sandwich without the bacon and Caesar dressing – try a dash of tzatziki instead. The Lamb on Pita is also a good low-fat option. Although it is no longer on the menu, it is possible to order a baked potato stuffed with spinach and feta, and served with a side salad.

Traditional Fare

❖ Order the Gammon Steak and Pineapple, the Beefeater or the Pork Medallions with a baked potato and steamed vegetables, or with a plain side salad. The Pansotti could be ordered with a tomato-based sauce, rather than the creamy sauce.

Desserts

❖ Try the Cherry Pavlova without the ice-cream.

MOZZARELLAS

Cape Town – Tyger Valley, Claremont,
Johannesburg – Melville, Isando, Rivonia
Pretoria – Hatfield

Mozzarellas offer Italian cuisine with flair, and take pride in using only fresh ingredients and producing all meals to order. Requests for low-fat cooking and preparation should not be too much of a problem. At the Claremont restaurant the manager suggested that, for larger groups, skim milk and other low-fat options could be ordered prior to your arrival.

Starters

❖ If you are planning to have a vegetarian main course, then the Carpaccio is a good starter, as long as you ask for a non-oil dressing.
❖ The Calamari can be dry-grilled on request, and ask for fresh lemon instead of the pesto.
❖ The Piccolo is an interestingly different low-fat starter.

Salads

❖ The Greek or House salads are served with dressings on the side.

Pasta

All pasta dishes can be served as half portions.
❖ The Alfredo can be ordered with the Napoletana sauce instead of the cream sauce.
❖ Calamari Arrabiatta is great as long as the calamari is dry-grilled.
❖ The Arrabiatta and Gnocchi are good low-fat options, while the Pasta Di Mare can be ordered with no cream.

Speciality Menu

All the following meals are served with pasta taken straight out of hot water (no extra oil added), and with steamed seasonal vegetables.

❖ The Vitello Diavolo is a perfect option, as is the Fillet Pizzaiola, which can be dry-grilled.

❖ The Fillet of Beef is a delicious choice, but remember to request no oil basting.

❖ Request no oil basting for the Free Range Chicken Breasts (avoid the herb lemon butter), the Calamari, the Catch of the Day and the Queen Prawns.

Pizza

❖ The pizzas on offer are very tasty with either half the cheese or even with no cheese at all – just piled high with vegetable toppings such as artichokes, sun-dried tomatoes, bell peppers, mushrooms, green peppers, etc. (*See* pages 183–184 for more advice on ordering pizzas.)

Desserts

❖ The Apple Pizza with no ice-cream or cream is a low-fat treat.

❖ Order a speciality coffee with no cream.

MUGG & BEAN

Cape Town – Waterfront, Durbanville
Johannesburg – Killarney Mall, South Johannesburg, Fourways, Balfour

The Mugg & Bean restaurants aim to offer you a variety of coffees of superior quality, served in a civilized atmosphere. You will be given a choice of either full-cream or fat-free milk, so you can happily embark on a guilt-free spree with teas, coffees, Milos, hot chocolates, café lattés, cappuccinos, etc.

Breakfasts

❖ Scrambled or poached eggs on toast (with no margarine) are not listed on the menu, but are available on request. Ask for fresh tomato or tomato sauce if you like.

❖ Eggs Royale or Eggs Benedict (with no hollandaise sauce) are low-fat treats – preferably served on fresh bread or plain, dry toast.

- Anchovy toast (with no butter) is a quick, easy option.
- If you want to avoid eggs, order the Mugg & Bean Health Breakfast, which includes yoghurt, muesli and fresh fruit.

On The Move & Quick And Easy
- A Giant Muffin is a meal in itself – have it plain or lightly spread with jam.
- A Toasted Ham and Tomato Sandwich can be ordered with no margarine.
- The Bagel with Lox – ordered with cottage cheese instead of cream cheese – and the Bagel with Brisket and Pickles are both good low-fat options.
- All the toasted sandwiches can be ordered with no margarine and even a chicken sandwich can be ordered without mayonnaise being used. I suggest smoked chicken and fresh tomato on whole-wheat toast.

Gourmet Sandwiches
All the sandwiches can be ordered with no margarine or mayonnaise.
- The Pastrami Reuben, Crab Roll on Baguette and Bagel Niçoise make for interesting sandwiches.
- The Roast Beef and Pickles on Rye is also a good option – remember to ask for no margarine and for plain salad instead of coleslaw.
- Order the Monte Christo Smoked Sandwich without mayonnaise.

Salads
- The Chinese Chicken Salad is a great choice, and is served with a delicious low-fat dressing.
- The Smoked Chicken Salad and House Salad can both be ordered without any dressing.

NANDO'S
In 1993 Nando's developed a 24-hour, toll-free care line, enabling customers to obtain a complete nutritional breakdown of any of their foods. The results of nutritional analysis have shown that, in general, all Nando's chicken products contain much less fat than other similar chicken products due to their specialized preparation and cooking methods.

Chicken Burgers

❖ All Nando's chicken burgers are made using filleted, skinless chicken breasts, which are grilled. The burgers make tasty, filling low-fat meals, as long as you remember to ask for no mayonnaise.

❖ If you are ordering an add-on, opt for a pineapple ring.

❖ The chicken in pita is also a filling yet healthy meal, and is served with salad – again, request no mayonnaise.

❖ The Prego Steak Roll without egg is another option.

Chicken Meals

❖ The Kebab on a roll is a delicious choice and can be served with salad instead of the chips.

Salads

❖ Nando's offers a Portuguese salad, with an option of added feta. The salad dressing is served separately, so it can easily be avoided. The salad and a Portuguese roll make a quick and simple light meal.

❖ The small coleslaw salad contains only 1.9 g of fat.

❖ Two recent additions to the salad selection are the Corn Salad and the Three-Bean Salad.

Sauces

❖ Most of the table sauces (mild, hot, extra hot, wild herb and garlic peri-peri) have a low fat content (3–4%), and can be used relatively freely to add extra zest to your meal.

OCEAN BASKET

There are approximately forty of these restaurants nationwide, and new branches are opening due to popular demand.

Starters

❖ The calamari stew, salad or curry are all made with calamari that has simply been boiled, and then just flavoured according to the requirements of the particular dish.

❖ Tzatziki and Taramasalata are also good starters.

❖ The pickled calamari heads have no added fat, so this makes a winning fat-free starter.

- The Village Salad is basically a Greek salad, and can be ordered with no dressing. The Fisherman's Salad, without dressing, is also a good choice.
- Oysters are another fat-free starter, which add zest to life without adding any inches to your waistline.
- For a hot starter, try the grilled calamari or Portuguese sardines.

Main Courses
- All the fish and seafood is grilled – ask for no lemon butter sauce to be used, as this is put on automatically (the tills are equipped with a special button to accommodate this request).
- Ask for steamed rice instead of chips and, again, ask for no lemon butter sauce to be used on the rice.

Desserts
- Kataifi or Baklava are both delicious, low-fat options – consisting mainly of phyllo pastry, nuts and honey.
- Galaktobouriko is similar to a milk tart, except that the pastry used is again phyllo – this makes it a suitable low-fat dessert.

O'HAGANS

There are currently about seventy O'Hagans restaurants nationwide. With the accent being on Irish pub fare, the food tends to be fairly wholesome and it tastes home-cooked. All the branches have standardized menus, which are updated regularly. Also, all branches are required to use low-fat mayonnaise and medium-fat margarine for cooking.

Starters or Light Meals
- Ostrich fillet slices, the smoked salmon, the Kerryman's tossed salad, the warm county chicken salad, the Greek salad or Stacey's smoked prawn and calamari salad are all good options. The salads are available in full or half portions – and use no dressings.

Main Meals
- House favourites include tasty but healthy options such as the vegetable, chicken or beef stir-fry. All meat and chicken used is lean and very little oil is used in the frying process.

- The O'Greek phyllo is a good choice for vegetarians, but request that the cheese sauce be left out.
- The venison casserole and lamb curry are great for cold nights, and the O'Kraut kassler with sauerkraut and mash as well as the steaks are also recommended. Avoid the creamy, cheesy sauces – opt for the monkey gland, peri-peri or barbecue sauces instead.
- Kilkee Kingklip is the fish dish with the lowest fat content. Most restaurants have proper grills under which you may request your fish to be grilled. Remember to ask for no lemon butter or other sauce – have fresh lemon instead. Order baked potatoes with cottage cheese, steamed rice or a small salad as an accompaniment.
- All vegetarian options are marked with a 'V' on the menu, but these dishes are not necessarily low in fat.

SPORTS CAFÉ

There are currently two Sports Cafés, one in Cape Town (at the Waterfront), and another in Gordon's Bay. Although visiting the Sports Café is very much a sporting experience, it does not count as a work-out – unfortunately! Luckily there are several great low-fat dishes on the menu, so it will not be necessary to guiltily run for the gym at the end of your meal.

The Greens Ana Gold
- The Olympic Greek Salad, Deep Sea Adventure and Chicken Run can all be served without dressings.
- If you are ordering the Gringo, ask for the chicken or beef to be sautéed without oil.

It's a Wrap
- The Thanksgiving Wrap is delicious even without the cheese.
- The Beef Lychee and Mango Wrap and the Smoked Chicken Wrap served just the way they are, will give you the edge over your competitors.

Sporting Le Coq
- The Birdie will give you a sporting chance – especially without the mayonnaise.

Snacking Side Out
❖ Try the Clubhouse without the bacon, and order a baked potato instead of chips.
❖ The Couch Potato, with a sweet and sour, honey and garlic, barbeque or peri-peri sauce, will help keep your shape from becoming like that of a potato!

Peak Pasta Performance
❖ The Raiders Roll-Up without the cheese is a tasty, energizing meal for people on the go.

Water Sports
❖ Ask for the Big Catch and the Blackened Fish to be grilled – not fried – served without the garlic and lemon butter.

Meat Is Meat And Bokke Must Eat
❖ The All Star Burger is a must for serious eaters, and all the steaks can be ordered dry-grilled with any of the same sauces used to accompany the Couch Potato (*see above*).

The Vegetable Patch
❖ Ask what the vegetables of the day are, and avoid fried vegetables and those with creamy sauces. Rather have one of the sauces offered with The Couch Potato (*see above*) – also to replace any cheese sauces – and add sour cream to your baked potato.

SPUR

Starters or Light Meals
❖ Devil's Fork Mushrooms are a mouthwatering, low-fat treat.
❖ The Spur baked potato – without butter – is a filling light meal, and remember that all branches of Spur have cottage cheese. Ask for no onion rings – order a salad garnish instead.
❖ The Salad Valley always offers a great variety. Go for the salads with no dressings – help yourself to some bread with cottage cheese, and add fresh fruit salad to make up a complete meal. Avoid the hot vegetables, unless you are told that they have been prepared by steaming only.

Main Meals

❖ A steak is a good choice, as long as you remember not to have meat more than three times a week. (*See* page 184 for general tips on ordering steaks.) Order the ladies' sirloin or fillet (200 g), or the Slimmers' steak, which is is served with salads from the Salad Valley.

❖ Choose your sauce from Monkey Gland, Mexican, Spanish, Texan-Chili, Peri-Peri or Spur's original BBQ sauce.

❖ The Spur Beef Sosatie is another good low-fat option, but make sure you have just half the sosatie and keep the other half for dinner the following night.

❖ The Hot Rock Rump (200 g) is a perfect choice as you get to cook your steak yourself, so you can be sure of no added fat. Order a baked potato and cottage cheese to go with it.

❖ If you are ordering a Chicken Burger, specify that it should be grilled, and that only BBQ sauce should be used – avoid other sauces.

❖ A Salad Burger can be ordered with any of the sauces mentioned above, with a large helping of salad (no dressing).

❖ A steak roll is also a good idea.

❖ If you are ordering the chicken kebab, ask for one of the two kebabs to be put in a doggy bag to be taken home.

❖ If you like fish, the catch of the day is usually a good choice. All Spurs are equipped with proper grills so that food can be grilled by heat from above, rather than on a heated grilling plate which may require fat being added.

STEERS

All beef burgers offered by Steers consist of 100% pure beef, and are flame-grilled using no oil. However, all the beef burgers are served with Thousand Island dressing, which has a high fat content. Similarly, all the chicken burgers are served with mayonnaise. If you are ordering a burger, therefore, remember to ask for no dressing to be used. If you are ordering a combo box, the chips can be replaced by adding extra salad and even a small, unbuttered cocktail roll.

Burgers

❖ If you are ordering a beef burger, go for the Steers Burger, Saucy Burger or Peri-Peri Burger (with no dressing).

❖ If you are ordering a chicken burger – which will be lower in fat than the beef burger – choose the plain Chicken Burger or the very tasty Tikka Chicken Burger (with no mayonnaise).

Speciality Rolls
❖ The Hero Steak Roll can be ordered with barbecue sauce only, leaving out the Thousand Island dressing and lemon oil basting.
❖ The Classic Ham and Cheese Roll can be made into a healthy meal by simply leaving out the mayonnaise and cheese.
❖ The Classic Tuna Salad Roll may be ordered with no mayonnaise and no butter on the roll.

Salads
❖ Order a fresh salad to go with your burger – instead of chips – and remember to specify that no dressing is to be used.

Desserts
❖ For dessert, a plain fruit salad will serve to enhance your mineral and vitamin intake, as well as satisfying your sweet tooth.

Sauces
The Steers Barbecue, Monkey Gland and Peri-Peri sauces are all fat free, and can be used to add flavour to your food either while you are eating at Steers or when you are preparing meals at home.

ST ELMO'S
St Elmo's branches are found nationwide in the form of restaurants, 'Pizzaways' or 'Sliceaways'. All their recipes are standardized, but the individual franchises do offer different degrees of flexibility – some will offer low-fat milk, for example, while others may not. You are sure to find a franchise near you where your particular needs can be met. I believe that it is always worth asking, no matter which restaurant you visit.

Starters or Light Meals
❖ A French salad is probably your safest starter option, unless you plan to have a vegetarian main meal, in which case the Greek, Niçoise, Italian or chicken salads are all suitable. At St Elmo's

avoiding salad dressing is easy, as the dressings for all the salads – except the Thai chicken salad – are served separately, to be added by patrons individually.

❖ At certain franchises the Thai chicken salad can be ordered with just a soy dressing, with no added cream or oil.

❖ The minestrone soup is perfect as a light meal. It is served with a mini pita bread, but remember to ask for low-oil pita bread.

Main Meals

❖ For general tips on ordering pizza, refer to the guidelines given on pages 183 and 184. The most suitable choices are the Casalinga, Deluca, Hawaiian, Regina or Hot Stuff – all with no mozzarella and just a sprinkling of feta. St Elmo's add no oil to their pizza bases. They do brush the edges of the pizza with oil as it comes out of the oven, though, but this procedure can be omitted on request.

❖ Most of the pasta dishes can be prepared without the use of cream. The Napoletana, Arrabiatta and tomato-based marinara pastas are all good options. The spinach and ricotta canneloni can be ordered with a tomato sauce. The chicken and mushroom gourmet pastas are also good options if ordered with no cream.

WANGTHAI

Thai Restaurant Holdings owns seven Asian restaurants nationwide, of which three are called Wangthai (in Cape Town, Sandton and Brooklyn, Pretoria). Two restaurants in the group are called Thaifoon (in Constantia and Tyger Valley), the others being Chai-Yo (Cape Town) and Saigon (Cape Town). Only Wangthai's menu has been considered here, although there are many similarities between the various menus.

Wangthai offers a wide variety of Royal Thai cuisines specially designed for the oriental palate and the more adventurous Westerner.

Starters (Appetizers)

❖ Meang Khum consists of a spinach cone filled with a variety of interesting ingredients. It is a very popular, tasty, low-fat starter.

❖ The Satay is another good option, preferably to be shared with a fellow diner.

Soups

❖ The mixed seafood soup with basil and the minced pork in glass noodle soup are both very tasty.

Main Dishes

❖ All the curries use a base of coconut cream, and are therefore best avoided. However, all the stir-fries can be dry-fried on top of the grill with no added oil if this is requested.

❖ The stir-fried beef in oyster sauce, beef with basil and chilli, and the stir-fried pork – either sweet and sour or with chilli paste – are all delicious options.

❖ The stir-fried chicken, either with basil and chilli or with cashew nuts, is a very popular and healthy choice.

❖ All the Thai salads are suitably low in fat.

❖ The steamed fish with lemon chilli sauce is a traditional meal with a very low fat content. The prawns with garlic and pepper – served in either tamarind or sweet and sour sauce – are also a low-fat but decadent option.

❖ For the vegetarian, it may be quite a dilemma choosing between the stir-fried mixed vegetables in soy sauce, the bean sprout stir-fry, and the mushroom stir-fry with cashews. All are delicious.

❖ If you are ordering any of the stir-fries just mentioned, ask for steamed rice or plain noodles with no oil. The other noodle dishes can be ordered as main meals, with no oil being used in the stir-frying process.

❖ One of the pleasures of dining in Thai restaurants is discovering new tastes and new dishes. If you succumb to the temptation of dishes that do not fall into the low-fat category, remember that most of the fat is usually contained in the sauce. Pick out the meat or vegetables, while leaving as much as possible of the sauce behind.

Desserts

❖ Although they may not be listed on the menu, Wangthai usually has a choice of refreshing fruit sorbets to choose from.

USEFUL ADDRESSES AND TELEPHONE NUMBERS

Association for Dietetics in South Africa (ADSA)
PO Box 1310
Cramerview
2060
Tel: (011) 886-8130
Fax: (011) 886-7612
E-mail: adsa@iafrica.com

Allergy Society of South Africa (ALLSA)
PO Box 88
Observatory
7935
Fax: (021) 448-0846

Cancer Association of South Africa (CANSA)
National Office:
PO Box 2121
Bedfordview
2008
Tel: (011) 616-7662
Fax: (011) 622-3424
Cancer Information Service:
Tel: 0800-22-6622 *(toll free)*

Food Advisory Consumer Service (FACS)
PO Box 72860
Lynnwood Ridge
0040
Tel/Fax: (012) 349-1448

Food Legislatory Advisory Group (FLAG)
The Directorate of Food Control
The Department of Health
Private Bag X828
Pretoria
0001
Tel: (012) 312-0511
Fax: (012) 312-0811

Health & Racquet Club
Head Office:
PO Box 379
Rondebosch
7701
Tel: (021) 710-8500

The Heart Foundation of Southern Africa
PO Box 15139
Vlaeberg
8018
Tel: (021) 510-6262
Fax: (021) 510-6267
Toll-free dietline: 0800-22-3222

Home Economics Association of Southern Africa (HEASA)
PO Box 29585
Sunnyside
Pretoria
0132
Tel: (012) 83-1844

Karen Protheroe – Registered Dieticians
PO Box 91
Constantia
7800
Tel: (021) 794-4269
E-mail address:
 karenrd@mweb.co.za

National Consumer Forum (NCF)
13 Berglelie Street
Winchester Hills Ext 3
Johannesburg
2091
Tel/Fax: (011) 680-4126

Packaging Council of South Africa (PACSA)
PO Box 782205
Sandton
2146
Tel: (011) 783-4782
Fax: (011) 883-7170

South African Association for Food Science and Technology (SAAFoST)
PO Box
17183
Congella
4013
Tel: (031) 261-6882
Fax: (031) 21-4124

South African Bureau of Standards
Private Bag X191
Pretoria
0001
Tel: (012) 428-7911

South African Diabetes Association (SADA)
PO Box 1715
Saxonwold
2132
Tel: (011) 788-4595
Fax: (011) 447-5100

South African National Consumer Union (SANCU)
PO Box 26242
Arcadia
0007
Tel/Fax: (012) 341-8158
Internet location:
http://africa.cis.co.za/consumer/
 main.html

South African Society for the Study of Obesity (SASO)
PO Box 930
Rivonia
2123
Tel: (011) 803-5375
Fax: (011) 803-2815

Vitamin Information Centre (VIC)
PO Box 182
Isando
1600

Index

Struik Publishers (Pty) Ltd
(a member of Struik New Holland Publishing (Pty) Ltd)
Cornelis Struik House
80 McKenzie Street
Cape Town 8001

Reg. No.: 54/00965/07

First published 1999

2 4 6 8 10 9 7 5 3 1

Project management by Linda de Villiers
Edited by Laura Milton
Designed and typeset by Lellyn Creamer
Cover design by Petal Palmer
Index by Gill Gordon

Reproduction of cover by Hirt & Carter, Cape (Pty) Ltd
Printed and bound by CTP Book Printers (Pty) Ltd,
Caxton Street, Parow 7500, Cape Town

ISBN 1 86872 403 4

DISCLAIMER

Every possible care has been taken in compiling this book. However,
the publishers and/or the authors cannot be held responsible for any
loss, damage or injury that occurs as a result of following the advice
contained herein. The health information in this book is not intended as
a substitute for a proper medical examination, or to replace the advice
of a registered dietician or medical doctor.